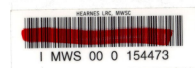

25.95

D0139851

The Loomis/Wood Model

DATE DUE

Demco

The Loomis/Wood Model
Applying Theory to Nursing Education, Research, and Practice

Maxine E. Loomis, D. Jean Wood,
Sandra S. Sweeney, and Joan Stehle Werner, Editors

National League for Nursing Press · New York
Pub. No. 15-2446

Copyright © 1992
National League for Nursing
350 Hudson Street, New York, NY 10014

ISBN 0-88737-540-5

The views expressed in this publication represent the views of
the authors and do not necessarily reflect the official views of
the National League for Nursing.

This book was set in Garamond by Pageworks. The editor and designer was Allan
Graubard. Automated Graphics Systems was the printer and binder.

The cover was designed by Lillian Welsh.

Printed in the United States of America

Contents

Contributors

Peggy L. Chinn, PhD, RN, FAAN, is an Associate Dean for Academics and Graduate Program Director, School of Nursing, University of Colorado, Denver, Colorado.

Karen Danielson, MSN, RN, is Assistant Professor, School of Nursing, University of Wisconsin-Eau Claire, Eau-Claire, Wisconsin.

Maxine E. Loomis, PhD, RNCS, FAAN, is Distinguished Professor Emeritus, College of Nursing, University of South Carolina, Columbia, South Carolina.

Winifred Morse, PhD, RN, is Associate Professor, School of Nursing, University of Wisconsin-Eau Claire, Eau-Claire, Wisconsin.

Sandra S. Sweeney, PhD, RN, is Professor, Department of Nursing Systems, University of Wisconsin-Eau Claire, Eau-Claire, Wisconsin.

Joan Steble Werner, is Professor, School of Nursing, University of Wisconsin-Eau Claire, Eau-Claire, Wisconsin.

D. Jean Wood, PhD, RN, is Professor, College of Nursing, University of South Carolina, Columbia, South Carolina.

Preface

We have written this book for baccalaureate and graduate level nurse clinicians, researchers, educators, and their students in nursing research and theory courses. Nursing care managers, special care nurses, and quality assurance coordinators should also find the ideas and examples presented here useful in conceptualizing and organizing their activities.

The book is presented in five major chapters. In Chapter 1, we explain the original development, refinement, and future directions of the Loomis/Wood Model. Emphasis is placed on the critique of this model for nursing research, education, practice, and theory development. Future directions for holistic nursing are emphasized. Chapter 2 contains an in-depth description of the application of the Loomis/Wood Model as an organizing framework for the undergraduate and graduate curricula at the University of Wisconsin-Eau Claire. Examples are given of the model's utility in medical model, nursing discipline, and nursing theory curricula. Research in which the Loomis/Wood Model was tested is reported in Chapter 3. Numerous examples are cited to illustrate the utility of the model with univariate and multivariate methods which examine actual and potential health problems, human response systems, and clinical decision making. Chapter 4 focuses on the clinical decision making, organizational activities, and specialty practice issues that can be clarified using the Loomis/Wood Model. Specific examples are cited in various health care settings and with the differing health care populations. A unique feature of this book is a concluding critique by Dr. Peggy L. Chinn, nurse scholar, futurist, activist, and editor of *Advances in Nursing Science.*

In an appendix, as well, we present the original article, "Cure: The Potential Outcome of Nursing Care," as published in *Image: The Journal of Nursing Scholarship,* in which the authors discuss the development and clinical utility of the model as originally conceived.

The Loomis/Wood Model is a framework—a structure for organizing information—and not a nursing theory. As such, it is only *one* way that has been found effective by some nurses; it is not *the* model that should be adopted by all nurses. The examples contained within this text illustrate the modifications that various clinicians, educators, researchers, and the authors have used in applying the model.

Our goal here is to demonstrate the utility of the Loomis/Wood Model for solving practical problems and providing new directions in nursing research, education, and practice. We hope to stimulate your thinking and expand your creative application of ideas within the discipline of nursing.

The Authors

1

Development, Refinement, and Future Directions of the Model

Maxine E. Loomis
D. Jean Wood

I deas embedded in the Loomis/Wood Model came from sources as diverse as shells along the shore—some known and some unknown. Each is valued, whether from the great inland lakes, Chicago's lake shore, the protected bays of New England, the roaring Pacific, or the rock tumbler beaches where South Carolina pushes and tugs with the Atlantic. There is no way to completely explain the act of nature that eventually emerges.

In this section, we have decided to present both the content and process of the emerging Loomis/Wood Model as we remember it. We write this in hopes that those attempting to utilize the model will be more forgiving if they understand its development, and more aggressive in their efforts to contribute to its further refinement. This chronology will undoubtedly offend some people by their inclusion and others by their exclusion. Students, colleagues, and friends have all influenced our thinking. We taught, thought, wrote, presented, listened; the feedback we received has been important to us. As prophets in our own country, we never lobbied for adoption of our ideas at Illinois or South Carolina. It took the efforts of Dr. Sweeney and Dr. Werner at the University of Wisconsin-Eau Claire to convince us we were on to something. The story goes like this.

THE BEGINNINGS

We arrived at the University of Illinois, College of Nursing, in January 1982, to join the new administrative team assembled by Dean Helen K. Grace. Despite the sub-zero temperatures and the horrors of commuting from the suburbs into the city every day, we were excited about our new roles as Director of the PhD Program (Maxine Loomis) and Chair of Psychiatric/Mental Health Nursing (Jean Wood). Never one to let snow collect under her feet, Dr. Grace scheduled a two-day administrative workshop in February to identify and plan a course of action for the college. As one might expect, this was more than just a team meeting to balance the budget. It was a think tank to stimulate our collective visions of what the college could contribute to the intellectual and practical development of the nursing profession.

One grand idea that emerged at the workshop was the responsibility for creating a nursing model that might provide a framework for curriculum development, practice, and research. *Nursing: A Social Policy Statement* (ANA, 1980) was fresh on our minds, and we were convinced we could make use of its wisdom to unite the diverse departments within the college and perhaps provide a model for the profession. Unfortunately, the dream remained just that: a dream. By May of 1982 Helen Grace had resigned her deanship to take a position with the W. K. Kellogg Foundation. It was not a good time for conceptual activity. In fact, the May 1982 faculty meeting was wrought with concerns about the developing model. "Are you saying we have to accept the ANA definition of nursing?" "Do we have these concepts in our curriculum?" "What about nursing diagnosis?" "What if our ideas don't fit with this model?" No resolution was achieved, and no process for resolution was identified. Time to drop back 20 yards and punt. While we received substantive input from individual faculty and graduate students regarding the utility of the model, there was no effort made to incorporate these ideas into the curricula of the college or the system as a whole. Perhaps ideas really do grow in small increments.

THE NEXT STEP

In 1983, Donna Diers, editor of *Image: The Journal of Nursing Scholarship*, issued a call for articles addressing practice theory. This seemed like an excellent opportunity to assure that the ideas that germinated in Chicago should not be lost. It was time to write (see Appendix).

We developed the idea of a cube that integrated clinical nursing, borrowed or derived theory, and nursing process. We found it somewhat more difficult, however, to explicate our conviction that good nursing care could actually cure patients. While our intent was to account for the complexities of practice theory in nursing, our ideas were reductionistic. With linear thinking a solid, significant component of each of our educations, a multivariate context was the best we had to offer; thus, the cube. The cube offered us a way to examine several variables simultaneously and suggest their interactions. It gave us a perspective on the practice of nursing, the contributions of related disciplines, and the nursing process. With the 1983 publication of our article, "Cure: The Potential Outcome of Nursing Care," we experienced the relief and satisfaction of seeing our ideas in print and waited for our colleagues to respond with further refinements of the proposed model.

Fall of 1984 found us at the University of South Carolina. Again, Jean Wood was to chair Psychiatric/Mental Health Nursing and Maxine Loomis was to guide the conception and delivery of a new PhD program in nursing science. By then our ideas had entered the open marketplace of scholarship and we were engaged in new challenges. If we could be criticized for anything at this point, it was that we had yet to promote the Loomis/Wood Model through workshops, publications, curriculum revision, and the like. Perhaps naively, we thought that ideas should sell themselves. In 1988, when Dr. Helen Erickson and a committee of committed faculty revised the baccalaureate curriculum at South Carolina, the Loomis/Wood Model was used as the conceptual framework. However, the model was downplayed and altered in the process to facilitate faculty acceptance of the end product. It was a humbling experience, to sit on the sidelines and not "interfere" with this process; however, personal pride can often interfere with the pragmatics of curriculum revision.

THE WISCONSIN CONNECTION

Unbeknown to us, the nursing faculty at University of Wisconsin-Eau Claire discovered our ideas as they revised their BSN and MS curricula. They requested that we come and consult. The Loomis/Wood Model was their conceptual framework, and faculty and clinical agencies were struggling with its implementation.

Our contacts with the faculty and clinicians in Eau Claire have been most rewarding. Their use of the Loomis/Wood Model is well documented in Chapters 2, 3, and 4. Our major contribution has been to encourage them to enjoy and capitalize on the theoretical and conceptual freedom offered by the model. We were convinced that it was important to foster a process whereby educators, clinicians, researchers, and theorists could utilize the model to develop their own ideas. The model was not prescriptive, but rather developmental, and it took this unique blend of nurses in Eau Claire, Wisconsin, to take advantage of the model's potential.

ELEMENTS OF THE MODEL

As originally proposed, the Loomis/Wood Model (1983) was atheoretical. The model's basic components were based on a definition of nursing (ANA, 1980), the organization of knowledge in the basic and social sciences, and the nursing process. It was designed to allow nurse educators, clinicians, researchers, and theorists to place their specific ideas within an integrated structure that allowed for both conceptual and empirical flexibility.

Nursing as "the diagnosis and treatment of human responses to actual or potential health problems" (ANA, 1980) provided the basis for development of categories down the left side of the model. In an attempt to clarify, yet keep things simple, four general types of situations with which nurses were likely to be concerned were outlined: (1) developmental life changes, (2) acute health deviations, (3) chronic health deviations, and (4) cultural/environmental stressors. The authors asserted that without the presence of at least one of these factors there is no actual or potential health problem.

Inherent in this approach, however, are two major problems. First, illness (or health problem) prevention and health promotion are not explicit but assumed. When caring for people experiencing any or all of these four circumstances, good nurses will be mindful of preventing further problems and promoting health. The original model and article, nor the definition of nursing upon which the model was based, do not sufficiently address this assumption. Subsequent iterations of the model to be presented later contain attempts to rectify this omission.

Second, and perhaps even more important, the model as originally designed and later refined is more reductionistic than holistic. The goal was to define people and their health care situations according to their component parts for the purpose of teaching and practicing nursing. While the model does not exclude the possibility of holism, it does not advocate it. This is an inherent flaw in any model that attempts to depict or specify variables and their relationships in a linear format. For example, when caring for a liver transplant patient the initial focus is likely to be the acute health deviations precipitated by a major intrusive and life-threatening procedure. As the immediate crisis resolves and healing occurs, the emphasis gradually shifts to the chronic nature of attending to a permanently altered health status. Medications, nutrition, daily activities, and regaining functional abilities become important topics. Of course, there is always the danger of an acute rejection or infection episode, liver biopsies, liver function studies, and similar events that require attention. Thus, acute episodes can and do occur during the course of a chronic health deviation.

In the meantime, transplant recipients are more than just a new liver. They are also experiencing developmental life changes related to their age and life situation. There is also a predictable period of time during which they are unable to resume normal roles as spouse, parent, or professional contributor, all of which can be very disruptive to the person and support system. Then there is the additional array of cultural/environmental life stressors. Births, deaths, hurricanes, organizational changes, and simply dealing with health providers and insurance companies increase the drama of daily life at a time when people have limited resources for coping. Someone, hopefully a primary nurse, needs to consider all of the above factors as a whole and not simply focus on SGPT or SGOT values to decide what assistance is required. The subcategories of actual or potential health problems must be identified as such and then integrated with the patient to create a complete picture of life and health for that person and significant others.

The human response system variables specified across the hori-

zontal axis of the original model (Loomis & Wood, 1983) suffer from
the same reductionistic limitations described above and for similar
reasons. An attempt was made to identify human response systems
according to the knowledge bases from which related information is
generated. The hope was that any nurse or student desiring relevant
information from the nursing and non-nursing sciences could readily
locate physical, emotional, cognitive, family, social, and cultural variables in textbooks and primary source materials. That is the way
information is currently organized. While these categories are not
mutually exclusive, they do not illustrate the contexts in which nurses
diagnose and treat patients. Until nursing develops and the world of
science adopts a taxonomy or classification system for the profession,
unrelated nomenclature will obfuscate rather than clarify the search
for information about human responses.

It is important to recognize that new developments in the physical,
behavioral, and social sciences often occur at the interface between
or among traditional fields of scientific endeavor. Such was the case
with biological engineering, human genetics, and psychoneuro-
immunology. While still reductionistic in their approach, these new
disciplines represent a synthesis of knowledge about response systems that must take place when dealing with *human* response systems. A holistic approach to the development of nursing science can
only enhance our understanding of the complex nature of human
responses and integrate them from fragmented systems into a
meaningful whole.

Original categories across the right third of the model include the
nurse and clients/recipients/patients in the clinical decision-making
process. Data collection, diagnosis, planning, treatment, and evaluation were selected as the relevant categories. It is important to recognize a major assumption not clearly presented in the original article
(Loomis & Wood, 1983): There is no data collection or "nursing
assessment" separate from the formulation of a nursing diagnosis.
While one might break down the process into more finite steps for a
course on clinical reasoning, the major operations involved are
nursing diagnosis, treatment, and evaluation. In this process, the
medical diagnosis is but one piece of relevant information.

For example, when working with people experiencing pain it is
important to know whether the pain is acute or chronic, possible
causes of the pain, and its impact on all human response systems. The
nurse and other health professionals must collect relevant data, accu-
rately diagnose problem areas, and plan interventions that require

both internal and external regulation. Frequent evaluation of the treatment(s), whether medication, relaxation, imagery, diversion, or some individualized technique, provide(s) feedback for further revision of the nursing diagnosis and treatment plan.

The clinical decision-making process utilized also depends on the theory of nursing selected by the faculty or administrators responsible for any given program. Given the emerging stage of theory development in nursing, the model was designed to allow for all possible choices and does not depend on any specific nursing or non-nursing theory. The assumption, however, is that choice of theory (Rogers, 1970; Andrews & Roy, 1986; Roy & Roberts, 1981; Levine, 1971)— adaptation, systems, self-regulation, or any others—will guide the collection of data, diagnosis, planning, treatment, and evaluation steps of the clinical decision-making process.

VARIATIONS ON A THEME

Only a few requests for reprints and speaking engagements following publication of "Cure: The Potential Outcome of Nursing Care" (Loomis & Wood, 1983) were forthcoming. In fact, the most sincerely positive and theoretically helpful responses came from our own graduate students and a national network of thoughtful nursing colleagues from whom we received critiques as well as compliments. This collaborative level of response has continued during the intervening nine years and has been most reinforcing. Our original intent was never to "sell" our ideas to a world starving for textbooks, manuals, and prescriptions for nursing research, practice, or education; nor is that our current interest. Ideas are meant to be tested and either developed, revised, adopted, or discarded. As mentioned earlier, the fact that the nurse clinicians, educators, and researchers in Eau Claire, Wisconsin, found our ideas so helpful has been at once humbling and stimulating. In the absence of a marketing campaign, they merely read an article and the ideas struck a chord.

As time passed and we had more opportunity to exchange ideas about the Loomis/Wood Model with students and colleagues, our original ideas changed and developed. What follows is a brief summary of the research, education, practice, and theoretical experiences that have helped change and re-shape our original model. We hope that an accurate reporting of these gradual shifts in thinking will not confuse, but rather stimulate additional model development.

Research: Classification Systems

In 1982, Maxine Loomis was asked to present a paper at the 1983 Forum on Doctoral Education in Nursing held at New York University. This paper, later published in *Nursing Research* (Loomis, 1985), was based on a content analysis of nursing dissertation abstracts and titles, 1976–1982. It provided an opportunity to apply the Loomis/ Wood Model to research of clinical nursing, to develop a parallel model for analysis of research of social issues in nursing, and to develop more specific definitions of the categories and subcategories within both models. The model for the study of clinical nursing (the original Loomis/Wood Model) was used to analyze all dissertations in which patients or patient analogs were among the study variables— in most cases the dependent variable.

A parallel model for the study of social issues in nursing was developed to analyze all of the dissertations in which nurses, nursing, or social issues were the objects of study. The categories were developed by reading the dissertation abstracts and consulting with nurses conducting research on social issues and placed in a cube format similar to the original Loomis/Wood Model (see Figure 1). Professional and policy issues were defined as questions relating to the knowledge base, learning, and science of nursing or a course of action adopted as expedient. The units of analysis in the study of social issues were identified as individual, group, organization, profession, culture, and nation, again reflecting the related disciplines from which nursing applies knowledge. The social decision-making process is the social/political equivalent of the nursing process (Rose, 1976).

Dissertations were identified as pertaining to either clinical nursing or social issues in nursing, and raters were instructed to check all subcategories that applied to each study. No limit was imposed on the number of categories or subcategories for any given study. Ratings were done by the investigator and two nursing doctoral student research assistants who were familiar with the models. Initial interrater agreement was 91.2%. The raters then met to resolve discrepancies and to further refine operational definitions within each model.

Results of the dissertation content analysis utilizing the clinical and social issues models are reported elsewhere (Loomis, 1985a, b); however, it is important to note that both models served the purpose of the analysis quite well. There were some interesting clusterings of

Figure 1
Model for the Study of Social Issues in Nursing

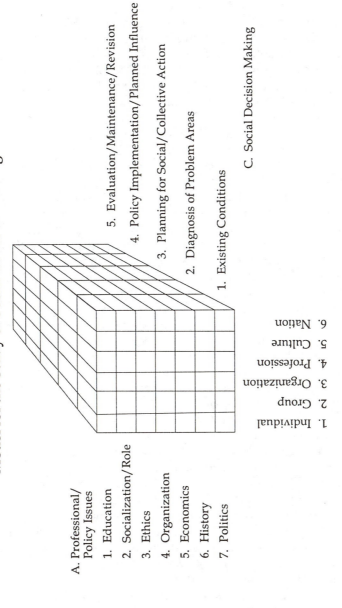

A. Professional/
Policy Issues

1. Education
2. Socialization/Role
3. Ethics
4. Organization
5. Economics
6. History
7. Politics

1. Individual
2. Group
3. Organization
4. Profession
5. Culture
6. Nation

B. Unit of Analysis

1. Existing Conditions
2. Diagnosis of Problem Areas
3. Planning for Social/Collective Action
4. Policy Implementation/Planned Influence
5. Evaluation/Maintenance/Revision

C. Social Decision Making

information which influenced subsequent development of both models which deserve discussion here.

Within the model for the study of clinical nursing, raters experienced periodic difficulty in distinguishing between the subcategories of actual and potential health problems. Pregnancy, for example, was rated as a developmental life change. Complicated pregnancy was rated as both a developmental life change and an acute health deviation. A study of toddlers with long-term tracheostomies measured acute and chronic health deviations as well as stressors and normal growth and development. This same multivariate approach is reflected in the data regarding human response systems studied. Nearly a quarter (24.8%) of the dissertations included both emotional and cognitive response systems, followed by physical and emotional (12.4%) and emotional and cognitive (11.2%) combinations. Thus, it is apparent that while the subcategories are defined as mutually exclusive, young investigators were conducting multivariate clinical studies which cross the distinctions contained in the definition of nursing and in the related knowledge disciplines.

The clinical decision-making category yielded somewhat predictable outcomes. Data collection and diagnosis were combined by many investigators (74.4%) conducting descriptive or qualitative studies. Intervention studies and quantitative investigators (23.4%) tended to combine the nursing process steps of treatment and evaluation in their design and data analysis. Therefore, for purposes of data analysis, the discrete clinical decision-making categories appear almost irrelevant. This same pattern was seen in the social decision-making category of the model for the study of social issues in nursing. Studies either utilized examination and diagnosis of problem area or policy implementation and evaluation in collecting and organizing their data. All of the above trends and difficulties were considered in subsequent refinement of the models.

In April, 1987, Maxine Loomis was asked to present a paper at the spring meeting of the Virginia/Carolina's Doctoral Consortium that would help the group move in the direction of identifying common conceptual research activities and interests across the member schools. The eventual goal of small group sessions to be held later in the meeting was to develop a system of research collaboration and networking that would support and enhance doctoral education in nursing. Preparation of this paper provided an excellent opportunity to synthesize prior thinking about the classification of nursing research (Roberts, 1954; Brown, 1958; Simmons & Henderson, 1964;

Abdellah, 1970; Notter, 1974; Gortner, Bloch, & Phillips, 1976; Gortner & Natum, 1977; Barnard & Neal, 1977; Ellis, 1977; Gunter & Miller, 1977; Highriter, 1977; Sills, 1977; O'Connell & Duffey, 1978) as well as more recent classification systems developed by Ozbolt et al. (1986) for University Microfilms International and that developed by Sigma Theta Tau for its Directory of Nursing Research (1987). This presentation was also the first time Donaldson and Crowley's (1978) seminal thinking about the discipline of nursing was incorporated into the original Loomis/Wood Model.

Our thoughts about the models for the study of clinical nursing and social issues in nursing were further expanded by contacts with the first three classes of PhD students in Nursing Science at the University of South Carolina, College of Nursing, Maxine Loomis's concurrent service on the ANA Cabinet for Nursing Research, and Jean Wood's leadership in initiating the Southern Nursing Research Society. It has become increasingly important over the past decade that the discipline of nursing responds to the challenge presented by Donaldson and Crowley (1978), Gortner (1975), Lindeman (1975), and McKay (1977) to develop a taxonomy that will organize knowledge within the profession. It is also important to recognize that the classification systems that follow in this section were designed to categorize nursing research. Debate continues regarding the wisdom or possibility of utilizing the same classification system for both research and practice, although one might hope the two would be related.

> *Research means to search or investigate thoroughly. It is a process of investigation or experimentation aimed at the discovery and interpretation of facts, the revision of accepted theories or laws in the light of new facts, or the practical application of such new or revised theories or laws. Research provides the bridge between the academic discipline of nursing science and the professional practice of nursing therapeutics. Research should be either theory testing or theory generating in nature, and this union of research and theory should provide the foundation for nursing practice. Research is therefore a logical place to begin the search for a system by which to organize nursing knowledge. (Loomis, 1989, p. 77)*

The model on which we are currently working and which was presented at the "Unity in Diversity" Nursing Research Conference sponsored by the American Nurses' Association Council of Nurse

Researchers in Chicago, Illinois, September 28, 1989 (see Figure 2), is
based on a series of new assumptions and definitions, and contains
different sets of variables from the original clinical and social issue
models. The primary definitional change is that of nursing itself, for
the examination of nursing science requires a definition that encompasses more than nursing practice. As such, *nursing is the science of
health and healing* which includes empirics or research, basic theory
development, and application or practice theory. Within this model,
clinical therapeutics is concerned with health-related human responses and nursing interventions as they apply to all client populations in all private and public settings. Social issues in nursing are
concerned with health-related responses which extend beyond the
individual and family or living unit.

The subcategories and variables outlined under clinical therapeutics and social issues can and have been used at a variety of national
and regional conferences to classify the research in which nurses are
engaged. Whether these categories are theoretically and practically
relevant is an empirical question. Details regarding the educational
and clinical expansion and application of this category system will be
presented later in this monograph.

Education: Curriculum Development

There is nothing so consuming of faculty time and energy as major
curriculum revision. Like weddings and funerals that tend to bring out
the best and worst in families, curriculum revision is guaranteed to
provide the stage on which nursing faculties can act out all of their
strengths and weaknesses, loves and resentments, trusts and fears.
Recognition of the vagaries of this process has led us to the somewhat
cynical conclusion that there is an inverse relationship between the
academic integrity of a nursing curriculum and the faculty's invest-
ment in political maneuvering and interpersonal drama. That's not to
say there are no theoretically sound curricula; however, they are few
and far between. Having offered that caveat, there are numerous
variations on the original Loomis/Wood Model and its subsequent
interactions that have been developed as models for nursing curricula.

One such successful curriculum is presented in detail by Sweeney,
Werner, Morse, and Danielson in this book. The University of Wisconsin–Eau Claire, School of Nursing, experience exemplifies what

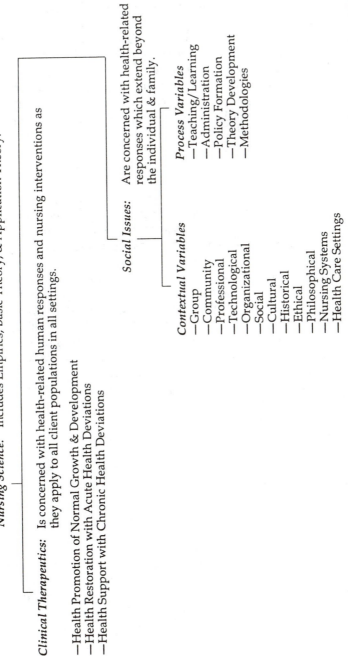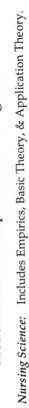

Figure 2
Model for the Development of Nursing Science

Nursing Science: Includes Empirics, Basic Theory, & Application Theory.

Clinical Therapeutics: Is concerned with health-related human responses and nursing interventions as they apply to all client populations in all settings.

—Health Promotion of Normal Growth & Development
—Health Restoration with Acute Health Deviations
—Health Support with Chronic Health Deviations

Social Issues: Are concerned with health-related responses which extend beyond the individual & family.

Contextual Variables
—Group
—Community
—Professional
—Technological
—Organizational
—Social
—Cultural
—Historical
—Ethical
—Philosophical
—Nursing Systems
—Health Care Settings

Process Variables
—Teaching/Learning
—Administration
—Policy Formation
—Theory Development
—Methodologies

can happen given thoughtful leadership and a faculty committed to working together for curricular change. Even then, the process was not without its bumps and bruises. As mentioned earlier, there were times when some faculty were frustrated that the Loomis/Wood Model was not more prescriptive of specific content; times when as consultants we felt like charlatans suggesting that if the faculty wanted to highlight or strengthen the family, community, or prevention components of their curriculum, we could work together to add the necessary variables to the original model. This process, however, gave all of us a clearer understanding of one of the strengths of the model—flexibility. While providing an overall structure—actual or potential health problems, human response systems, and clinical decision making—the model does not dictate specific content, nor does it even require use of the originally proposed subcategories. It does, however, allow faculty to focus more on curriculum content than model building—at best a risky process for a bright, diverse collection of nurses with advanced degrees.

For example, during the past seven years we have consulted with one faculty whose traditional approach to undergraduate curriculum clearly included the right of protecting and preserving ones "property." While talking about integration and holistic nursing, the undercurrent of med-surg, psych, peds, OB, and community prerogatives could not be ignored. They made the model work for them by adopting the structural elements in Figure 3.

Another approach to altering the model for a faculty that did not want to directly emphasize nursing process, but saw clinical decision making as a strand that ran throughout the curriculum, is contained in Figure 4. This model relates three generic human responses with their general category of nursing intervention and reflects the faculty's commitment to client populations (individual, interpersonal/family, and cultural/environmental groupings). In this curriculum, the system of health care delivery is emphasized in course content more than the nursing process along the third dimension of the cube. This faculty made this model work for their students and faculty in their clinical settings, and that's what was important.

At the time of this writing, the authors tend to favor different model elements depending on the level of student and the program outcome objectives. We remain committed to the use of two parallel models—one for clinical therapeutics and another for social issues in nursing. At the baccalaureate level, clinical therapeutics should be placed in the foreground with social issues as a consistent backdrop, while at

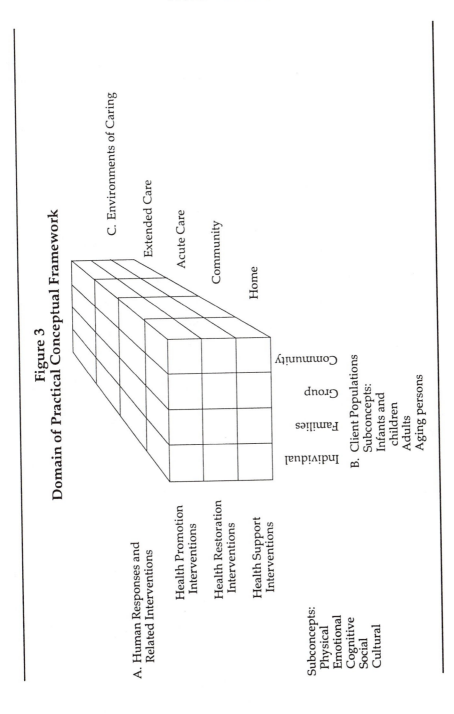

Figure 3
Domain of Practical Conceptual Framework

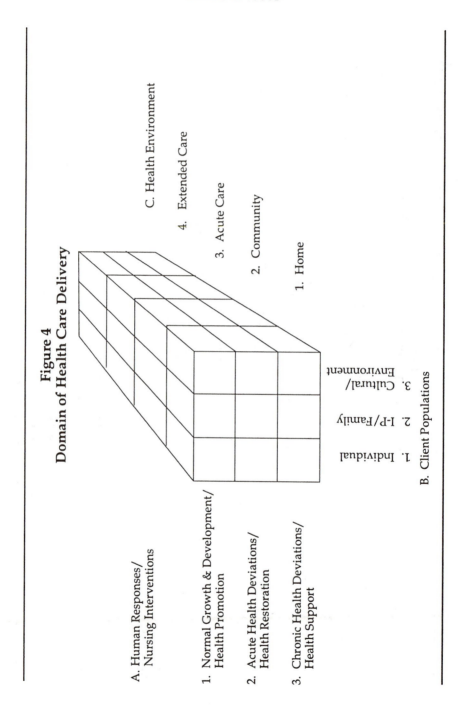

Figure 4
Domain of Health Care Delivery

C. Health Environment
4. Extended Care
3. Acute Care
2. Community
1. Home

3. Cultural/Environment
2. I-P/Family
1. Individual
B. Client Populations

A. Human Responses/Nursing Interventions
1. Normal Growth & Development/Health Promotion
2. Acute Health Deviations/Health Restoration
3. Chronic Health Deviations/Health Support

the master's degree level both clinical therapeutics and social issues should receive equal attentions. At the doctoral level, the content and process of education should shift primarily to Figure 2 and the development of nursing science.

It is not likely that every nursing degree program regardless of educational level will choose to equally emphasize all elements of either the clinical therapeutics or social issues models. For example, the model represented in Figure 5 was designed with a faculty that was committed to objectives linking general types of human responses with types of nursing intervention. They and their clinical settings were further committed to examining health and health care across the lifespan within the family or living unit context, and their undergraduate students were expected to implement the nursing process within the strengths and limitations of the person's health environment.

The contextual variables, health issues, and process variables within the social issues provided the background for baccalaureate graduates who would be delivering direct professional nursing care as illustrated in Figure 6. It is interesting to note that this particular faculty chose not to prescribe specific health issues within the social issues model in Figure 6. Faculty teaching the issues course, and all other courses, were encouraged to identify timely, relevant health issues related to their course content and remain flexible from one semester to the next.

At the master's degree level, this same faculty provided guidance for advanced students to select an area of clinical specialization within the parameters of their faculty strengths represented in Figure 5. Because the graduates of the master's program would assume positions of clinical and administrative leadership within the health care system, clinical therapeutics and social issues were balanced in the program objectives. Nursing theories, derived theories, and research methods were stressed as the foundation for advanced practice.

These brief examples are presented to offer some idea of the curriculum options available when using the clinical and social issues models. Nursing faculties can select the nursing theories or theory as well as the derived theory (theories) that best fit with their expertise and available clinical settings and populations while addressing nursing's metaparadigm of *person, health, environment,* and *nursing* (Fawcett, 1984). Chapter 2 of this book contains a much more detailed example of curriculum innovation by the nursing faculty at the Uni-

Figure 5
Human Response and Nursing Intervention Emphasis

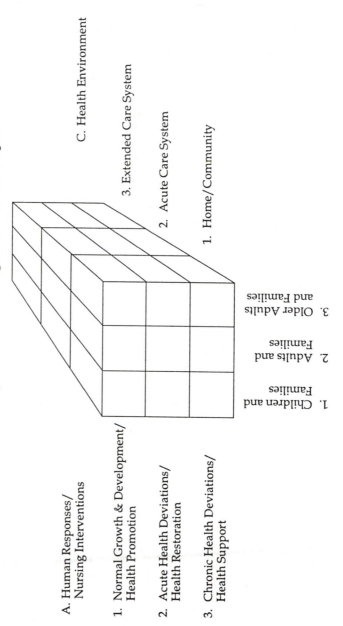

A. Human Responses/
Nursing Interventions

1. Normal Growth & Development/
Health Promotion

2. Acute Health Deviations/
Health Restoration

3. Chronic Health Deviations/
Health Support

1. Children and Families

2. Adults and Families

3. Older Adults and Families

B. Client Populations

1. Home/Community

2. Acute Care System

3. Extended Care System

C. Health Environment

Figure 6
Curriculum Emphasis on Social Issues

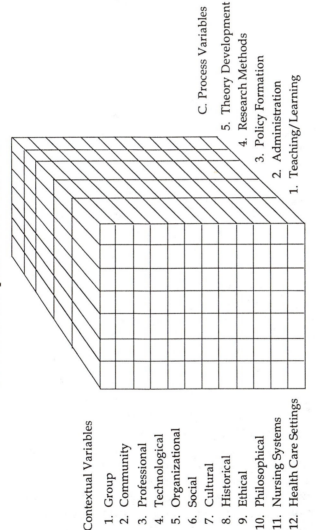

A. Contextual Variables

1. Group
2. Community
3. Professional
4. Technological
5. Organizational
6. Social
7. Cultural
8. Historical
9. Ethical
10. Philosophical
11. Nursing Systems
12. Health Care Settings

B. Health Issues

C. Process Variables

5. Theory Development
4. Research Methods
3. Policy Formation
2. Administration
1. Teaching/Learning

versity of Wisconsin-Eau Claire using the original Loomis/Wood Model (1983). They were among the first to teach us about the flexibility and potential of ideas, even after they are committed to writing.

Practice: Health Care Prototypes

It is important to highlight a neglected but important aspect of the Loomis/Wood Model—the four prototypes of health care situations. These prototypes are important because they provide nurses with the opportunity to break out of the cause and effect, linear reasoning model which has contributed to a reductionistic rather than holistic approach to health care. What was proposed are four types of health care situations:

1. Health problems precede human responses.
2. Human responses precede health problems.
3. Health problems are defined by human responses.
4. Health problems interact with human responses.

Specific examples of each of these prototypes are contained in the original article and will not be repeated here (see Appendix). However, it is important to emphasize their significance in displacing the linear, cause and effect, approach to nursing care. We don't really know what "causes" health problems. At best we can document that one event precedes another, but that does not necessarily imply causality; it merely identifies a point in time to which one attends. This is the case with most acute health problems.

In acute situations, the onset of illness is usually recorded as the time when symptoms were noticed, when the person requested health care assistance, or when an accident or traumatic event occurred. A youngster falls from a backyard swing and is taken to the local emergency room for treatment of a broken arm. Members of a family vacationing by the ocean each begin to develop symptoms of nausea, vomiting, diarrhea, and lethargy, and the search is on for the possible cause of food poisoning or tainted seafood. An executive finally retires from the "corporate rat race" with visions of golf, travel, and relaxation firmly planted by his wife, only to be admitted to a coronary care unit six months later complaining of chest pain. At first glance, all of these situations are deceptively simple. When viewed through the lens which focuses on acute care, these health problems precede certain predictable human responses.

The youngster with a broken arm will need to adjust to certain limitations for four to six weeks, and care of this time-limited health problem will also require adjustments on the part of parents, family, and friends. Likewise with the vacationing family. Once there is a determination of probable cause and the threat to life is minimized or negated, they can look forward to a mild disruption in their original plans for the week and a return to "normal" activities. Even the retired executive is likely to be discharged within a week with a prescription for diet, physical activities, and perhaps medication or directions to stop smoking. After some adjustments in lifestyle, he and his wife can get on with their retirement. However, is there really anything that makes these three situations any different from those in which human responses precede health problems?

The difference between prototypes one and two appears to be merely a matter of timing and focus. Because of the episodic nature of health care, there is a tendency to attend to the acute problem and its relief. If these patients and significant others are lucky, there will be nurses available who can also assist in planning for and dealing with the human responses related to an eight-year old with a casted arm, nutritional needs following dehydration, or lifestyle changes following a mild myocardial infarction. But what would happen differently if the focus of care also included the human responses which preceded the acute health problem?

For example, what if the nurse in the emergency room knew that the youngster with the broken arm was being punished for hitting his younger sister and was not to be out of his room when the accident occurred on the swing? What if the vacationing family had been travelling together for the first time since their father's re-marriage following the mother's death only one year earlier? And what if the executive had been forced to take early retirement in the midst of a corporate reorganization? Since human responses are merely behaviors (physiological, psychological, cognitive, and motor) that are always occurring, it is often difficult to determine what is stimulus and what is response. While it is temporally possible to produce a chronology of what precedes what, even that activity is distorted by the point in time one selects for beginning the explanation.

Health care prototypes three and four serve to further complicate the development of mutually exclusive categories. Situations in which health problems are defined by human responses are readily available in nursing, psychiatry/psychology, and even general medicine. Examples from the approved NANDA nursing diagnostic categories (NANDA, 1989) will be used here to illustrate the complex nature of nursing practice despite the development of a clear set of definitions and guidelines.

All of the NANDA-Approved Nursing Diagnoses (NANDA, 1989) include a definition of the diagnosis, defining characteristics, and related factors. For example, one possible nursing diagnosis for the family whose eight-year old has a broken arm might be Parental Role Conflict. Parental Role Conflict is defined as "The state in which a parent experiences role confusion and conflict in response to crises" (p. 57). Defining characteristics for this diagnosis include parental expression of inadequacy to provide for the child's physical and emotional needs as well as demonstrated disruption in parental role. While the NANDA Taxonomy labels these behaviors as defining characteristics of the diagnosis, they might also be regarded as human responses, in which case the health problem is defined by the human responses. Logic suggests that intervention and amelioration of the human responses, by definition, removes or cures the health problem.

Likewise, the retired husband and wife referred to earlier might receive the nursing diagnosis of Altered Health Maintenance upon his immediate return from the hospital. Their "Inability to identify, manage, and/or seek out help to maintain health" (NANDA, 1989, p. 77) could be demonstrated by their inability to take responsibility for basic health practices related to his cardiac status and expressed interest in improving their health behaviors. Following health teaching and nursing assistance, with daily health management there should be a marked improvement in this couple's self-care human responses, and if so, no need for retaining the original diagnosis of a health or nursing care problem.

The above conceptual difficulties with health care prototypes one, two, and three might lead to the conclusion that prototype four, in which health problems interact with human responses, is the most reasonable conceptual approach to defining the holistic experience of health and illness. That appears to be a parsimonious conclusion until one considers the separations inherent in this last category. First, as originally presented, prototype four has been utilized to examine the ongoing nature of chronic health problems. These are problems or conditions which require attention every day of one's life and for which there is no reasonable expectation of "cure," such as multiple sclerosis, arthritis, diabetes, or hypertension. However, chronic health problems each provide unique patterns of remissions and exacerbations (acute episodes) and persons with chronic conditions also experience acute problems such as influenza, broken bones, and life crises.

Second, and perhaps more importantly, there is no way to clearly, cleanly separate "health problems" and "human responses" within a holistic approach to working with real people. In fact, health problems are also human responses and human responses are health problems from a holistic perspective. The two are inseparable!

FUTURE DIRECTIONS

By now the reader may ask, "What are we supposed to do now that you've raised concerns about the Loomis/Wood Model and the health care prototypes?" Unfortunately, those questions occurred to us as we wrote this chapter. The only answer we can offer is to use this model for what it is: a vehicle for describing nursing practice, research, and education as they currently exist in many settings. Be creative and enjoy its flexibility. Develop new variations that better suit your needs and concerns. And don't expect something prescriptive that was not intended in the original model.

The original Loomis/Wood Model was based on the ANA (1980) definition of nursing as "the diagnosis and treatment of human responses to actual or potential health problems" and was weighted toward a problem or illness orientation. That doesn't mean that health promotion cannot be included. Because the original model was designed to separate the whole into its component parts for purposes of analysis and teaching, there has been a tendency to dismiss it as reductionistic rather than holistic. However, the model can also be viewed as a highly operational expression of contemporary thinking about nursing. New models must be developed to address some of the philosophical and definitional issues yet to be resolved.

Hall and Allan (1986) have proposed a definition of nursing that acknowledges the two distinct realms of illness and health: "Nursing is concerned with the phenomena of human responses to illness and health." They go on to assert that the disease and the health models cannot coexist within nursing unless we develop two distinct professions. Schlotfeldt (1987) went even further in her proposed definition of nursing as "the appraisal and the enhancement of the health status, health assets, and health potentials of human beings." Schlotfeldt's definition focuses the profession entirely on health. In a panel discussion at the 1987 Nurse Theorist Conference in Pittsburgh, Leininger predicted the fading out of nursing diagnosis by the year 2000. As she stated (cited in Smith, 1988), "We will get our best kind of taxonomy when we know our unique dimensions and substantive knowledge by which we will then order and classify. We are still in a rich exploratory open phase of study." Her caveat suggests a definitive movement away from the problem and illness focus that has been the driving force of our health care and reimbursement system for so long. This is the system on which the ANA (1980) definition of nursing and the Loomis/Wood Model was based.

While we would applaud a more holistic, health-oriented approach to nursing practice, research, and education, we do not consider such a revolution possible by the year 2000. We will work toward a more humanistic advancement of the profession while maintaining a realistic foundation in the system that is reality for the majority of nurses and patients. The Loomis/Wood Model is not a theory for health care revolution. It is a model of what is and what could be accomplished by small, thoughtful increments.

REFERENCES

Abdellah, F. G. (1970). Overview of nursing research, 1955–1968, parts 1, 2, and 3. *Nursing Research, 19,* 6–17, 151–162, 239–252.

American Nurses' Association (1980). *Nursing: A social policy statement.* Kansas City, MO: The Association.

Andrews, H. A., & Roy, C. (1986). *Essentials of the Roy adaptation model.* Norwalk, CT: Appleton-Century-Crofts.

Barnard, K. E., & Neal, M. V. (1977). Maternal-child nursing research: review of the past and strategies for the future. *Nursing Research, 26,* 193.

Brown, A. F. (1958). *Research in nursing,* Philadelphia: W. B. Saunders, Co.

Donaldson, S. K., & Crowley, D. M. (1978). The discipline of nursing. *Nursing Outlook, 26,* 113.

Ellis, R. (1977). Fallibilities, fragments and frames: Contemplation on 25 years of research in medical-surgical nursing. *Nursing Research, 26,* 177.

Fawcett, J. (1984). The metaparadigm of nursing: Present status and future refinements. *Image: The Journal of Nursing Scholarship, 16*(3), 84–87.

Gortner, S. R., Bloch, D., & Phillips, T. R. (1976, March-April), Contributions of nursing research to patient care. *Journal of Nursing Administration*, 26.

Gortner, S. R., & Nahm, H. E. (1977). An overview of nursing research in the United States. *Nursing Research, 26*, 10.

Gould, S. J. *The Mismeasure of man.* New York: W. W. Norton, 21.

Gunter, L. M., & Miller, J. C. (1977). Toward a nursing gerontology, *Nursing Research, 26*, 208.

Hall, B. A., & Allen, J. D. (1986). Sharpening nursing's focus by focusing on health, *Nursing and Health Care, 7*(6), 315.

Highriter, M. E. (1977). The status of community health nursing research, *Nursing Research, 26*, 183.

Levine, M. E. (1971). Holistic nursing. *Nursing Clinics of North America, 6*(2), 258–263.

Loomis, M. E. (1985a). Emerging content in nursing: An analysis of dissertation abstracts and titles—1976–1982. *Nursing Research, 34*, 113.

Loomis, M. E. (1985b). Emerging nursing knowledge. In J. C. McCloskey & M. K. Grace (Eds.), *Current Issues in Nursing,* 2nd ed. Boston: Blackwell Scientific Publications.

Loomis, M. E., & Wood, D. J. (1983). Cure: The potential outcome of nursing care. *Image: The Journal of Nursing Scholarship, 15*(1), 4.

Loomis, M. E. (1989, September). *Historical overview: Comparison of nursing research classification systems.* Paper presented at the ANA, Council of Nurse Researchers, Chicago, Illinois.

Notter, L. E. (1974). *Essentials of Nursing Research.* New York: Springer.

O'Connell, K. A., & Duffey, M. (1978). Research in nursing practice: Its present scope. In N. C. Chaska (Ed.), *The nursing profession: Views through the mist.* New York: McGraw-Hill.

Roberts, M. M. (1954). *American nursing: History and interpretation.* New York: Macmillan.

Rogers, M. (1970). *Theoretical basis for nursing.* Philadelphia: F. A. Davis.

Rose, R. (1976). *The dynamics of public policy.* Beverly Hills, CA: Sage.

Roy, C., & Roberts, S. (1981). *Theory construction in nursing: An adaptation model.* Englewood Cliffs, NJ: Prentice-Hall.

Schlotfeldt, R. M. (1967). Defining nursing: A historic controversy. *Nursing Research, 36*, 64.

Sigma Theta Tau International. (1987). *Directory of nurse researchers.* Indianapolis: The Association.

Sills, G. M. (1977). Research in the field of psychiatric nursing. *Nursing Research, 26*, 201.

Simmons, L. W., & Henderson, V. (1964). *Nursing research: Survey and assessment.* New York: Appleton-Century-Crofts.

Smith, M. J. (1988). Perspectives on nursing science. *Nursing Science Quarterly, 2*, 80–85.

2

Application and Utilization of the Loomis/ Wood Model as the Conceptual Framework for Curriculum Design

Sandra S. Sweeney
Joan Stehle Werner
Winifred Morse
Karen Danielson

*N*urse educators in the United States can trace their concern for providing students with quality programs of instruction to the early decades of this century. M. Adelaide Nutting, who chaired the committee responsible for authoring the report "The Educational Status of Nursing," is often credited with the professions' initial efforts to improve the caliber of nursing education programs. This initial effort to describe the status of nursing education in the United States may have failed to quickly generate significant changes in the "appalling" practices described. However, it did serve to establish nursing as a profession and confirmed the need to continue investigations regarding educational practices used to teach both knowledge and skills to students enrolled in various nursing curricula (Kelly, 1985).

The Goldmark (1923) report, published some nine years later, more clearly characterized some of the specific problems facing nursing education in America. Common concerns identified by this committee included poor admission and selection standards for students, inadequately prepared faculty, and erratic programs of formal instruction that often neglected meeting the instructional needs of the students whenever meeting the needs of the hospital was deemed to be more important (Kelly, 1985).

Since these early struggles, nurse educators have labored to improve, standardize, and cultivate superior educational programs of nursing. These efforts, combined with the profession's acceptance of voluntary accreditation provided by the National League for Nursing, ensure the delivery of high-quality programs of instruction. Recently, however, concerns have arisen that the earlier efforts to ensure quality education have been displaced by preoccupation with the delineation of theoretical, conceptual, or organizing frameworks whose purpose is to illustrate the curricular structure and function of each school of nursing's approach to the discipline. Indeed, the criteria governing the accreditation process includes as its first requirement under the section titled "Curriculum" . . . the need for faculty to demonstrate that curriculum is "logically organized, internally consistent and reflects the mission and/or beliefs of the nursing unit" (National League for Nursing, 1985, p. 13).

While schools of nursing can operate fully with only the approval of a state board of nursing, receiving full accreditation status by the National League for Nursing substantially improves the credibility of the school. Indeed, the National League for Nursing has long been recognized as the steward responsible for ensuring and maintaining the quality of institutionalized educational programs of nursing— regardless of the degree being offered: diploma, associate degree, bachelor's, or master's. Thus, most schools of nursing strive to attain and maintain their accreditation status by this auspicious body.

The need to document and periodically revise a logically organized and internally consistent curricular framework often requires an inordinate and unnecessary commitment of time, energy, and effort on the part of numerous faculty members. It is, indeed, a difficult task to ensure that the curriculum framework is sufficiently organized so that it contains up-to-date content from a variety of related disciplines as well as accommodating the continually evolving perspectives of contemporary nursing. Finally, the curricular framework must also meet the requirements of logic and consistency with the institution's articulated mission, philosophy, and belief statements.

For the most part, nurse educators have accepted as valid many of the educational practices recommended by curriculum theorists as being directly applicable to planning and implementing nursing curricula. Chater (1975) defined "a conceptual framework as a structure for supporting, defining, and enclosing selected parts for a larger cohesive whole. Thus, the development of a curricular framework is a highly complex decision-making process involving numerous choices" and organizing them such that "one sees the parts in relation to each other while discarding the parts that do not fit into the enclosing structure" (p. 429). The Chater (1975) model proposed only three components to construct a conceptual framework adequate to support a nursing curriculum: students, settings, and subjects.

Torres and Stanton (1982) argue the conceptual framework must be deduced from the curriculum philosophy. Whether or not the curricular framework is derived from the school's statement of philosophy is perhaps not as important as the extent to which it serves to identify the content of the curriculum and the logical and sequential nature of the content as it progresses throughout each of the program's components. Bevis (1982) provides one of the clearest and most comprehensive definitions of what a conceptual framework should be when she states: "A conceptual framework is an interrelated system of premises that provides guidelines or ground rules for making all curricular decisions—objectives, content, implementation, and evaluation." The conceptual framework is the "conceptualization and articulation of concepts, facts, propositions, postulates, theories, phenomena, and variables relevant to a specific nursing educational system" (p. 26). Thus, the framework becomes a dynamic document, subject to alteration as the generation of knowledge, conditions of practice, qualifications of faculty, and society change. Regardless of how one chooses to define the general idea of conceptual framework, there does seem to be some agreement as to its role in specifying both the content to be taught and the structure within which the content will be sequenced.

The search for the "perfect framework," one that meets Bevis's (1982, 1989) criteria in that it allows for continuous revision and yet remains sound and intact, continues as a goal of many nurse educators. Some might suggest such an ideal framework does not exist. This chapter challenges those assertions and illustrates how one model—the Loomis/Wood Model for Clinical Nursing (Loomis & Wood, 1983)—can provide a flexible, logical, and consistent organizing framework compatible with a wide range of nursing curricula and capable of easily adapting to diverse mission statements, disparate philosophies, and continually changing knowledge.

Previously, an analysis of conceptual frameworks conducted by Santora (1980) indicated undergraduate and graduate nursing educational programs tended to have theoretical, conceptual, or organizing frameworks that fit into six general albeit different categories: (1) none, (2) ambiguous, (3) multiple, (4) adaptation, (5) systems, and (6) developmental. In addition, nurse educators have also incorporated frameworks developed by nurse theorists as another means of organizing their curricula. Regardless of the framework selected, however, their range of usefulness has generally been controlled and confined to the particular phenomena that are explicated within the specific conceptual or theoretical core. The Loomis/Wood Model, however, provides nurse educators with a precise yet abstract framework tangible enough to allow the integration of content from nursing's related disciplines, as well as the ever expanding and changing knowledge base of the discipline itself. The Loomis/Wood Model makes it possible and feasible for nurse educators to adapt and revise both the content and processes of a nursing curriculum while keeping the original organizing structure intact and unchanged.

The Loomis/Wood Model first appeared in the nursing literature in *Image: The Journal of Nursing Scholarship* in 1983 (Loomis & Wood, 1983). The original work has been reprinted in the appendix of this publication. Admittedly, the model's application to specific aspects of nurse education, research, and practice has been limited to date. Yet, what applications have been made have been remarkably accurate and valid. Thus, it would appear that the model has been able to adequately demonstrate its ability to meet the critical test of substantiating its utility given particular situations and needs.

In addition to the flexibility provided by an abstract model, the Loomis/Wood Model also incorporates and builds upon: (1) a nationally accepted definition of nursing; (2) the nursing diagnosis taxonomy; (3) a multivariate system of information processing and decision making; and (4) relationships among three discrete components perceived germane to the professional practice of nursing—actual or potential health problems, human responses, and nursing clinical decision making (see Figure 1). Another unique dimension of the model is that it explicates four specific prototypes of health care situations which nurse educators, researchers, or practitioners can

Figure 1
Model for the Study of Clinical Nursing

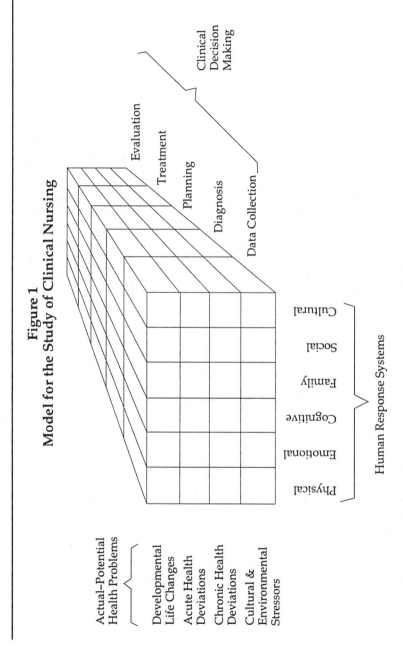

Clinical Decision Making

Evaluation
Treatment
Planning
Diagnosis
Data Collection

Cultural
Social
Family
Cognitive
Emotional
Physical

Human Response Systems

Actual-Potential Health Problems

Developmental Life Changes
Acute Health Deviations
Chronic Health Deviations
Cultural & Environmental Stressors

From "Cure: The Potential Outcome of Nursing Care," by M. Loomis and D. Wood, *Image 15*, p. 4. Reprinted by permission.

use to ascertain the appropriate role(s) for nursing contrasted with those accorded medicine. These prototypes also assist in determining and prioritizing treatment modalities commensurate with the number and system of human responses affected, and clearly separate the focus and substance of nursing interventions from those ascribed to practitioners of medicine. Thus, the model provides direction upon which both the structure and syntax of nursing can be constructed and operationalized.

How can the Loomis/Wood Model be used as a curricular organizing framework? How can it be employed to illustrate and interpret a variety of borrowed or unique theoretical and conceptual frameworks currently used to guide nursing educational programs? One logical beginning might originate with the faculty's decision to initiate their curricular planning efforts with one of the three major dimensions of the model: (1) Actual/Potential Health Problems; (2) Human Response Systems; or (3) Clinical Nursing Decision Making. Once this decision has been made, subsequent planning regarding the organization and sequencing of content becomes a reflection of the specific dimension selected to serve as the curriculum's primary focus by the faculty. Perhaps the following vignettes can illustrate some of the model's flexibility using distinctly different foci as comprising the principal theme.

A NURSING CURRICULUM BASED ON "THE MEDICAL MODEL"

Historically, many nursing curricula have patterned their educational programs and course content following traditional medically based subject areas. Thus, nursing students learned the theory and practice of medical, surgical, maternity, pediatric, and psychiatric nursing. While such an organizing framework would no doubt raise questions among many of today's nurse educators, such a curriculum could, if desired, be operationalized using the Loomis/Wood Model. For example, nursing courses could be organized according to the theme of Acute or Chronic Health Deviations. The deviations in health could be easily grouped according to traditional disease-oriented clusters. The roles of physician/nurse would most probably follow the Loomis/Wood Model's first prototype of health care situations in which human problems precede human responses—thus, the medical role would remain fundamental and the nurse would be expected to function collaboratively targeting his or her nursing efforts toward stabilizing the patient while trying to assist the physician in curing/ treating the disease. Obviously, in this type of curriculum, nursing interventions would be planned to complement the medical regime of treatment. Content could be further organized employing any one of several related themes, such as patterns of human development, stress-adaptation, or health-illness, or moving from simple to complex health deviations. The definitions of nursing contained in the Loomis/Wood Model could remain applicable, although any utilization of the nursing diagnosis taxonomy may need to focus on those nursing diagnoses that are more medically oriented.

A NURSING CURRICULUM BASED ON "NURSING AS A DISCIPLINE MODEL"

Perhaps the notion of creating a nursing curriculum using concepts and theories generated from nursing's existing field of knowledge may appear as remote to many nurse educators as the preceding example using the medical model, albeit for different reasons. The major challenge confronting curriculum planners utilizing a discipline of nursing approach rests with their ability to document an adequate number of research-based investigations currently extant in which nursing knowledge and practice have been clearly identified and validly and reliably tested. While many nurse educators might voice concern over the prematurity of this type of a curriculum, the Loomis/ Wood Model is capable of accommodating such an endeavor if and when it might be deemed feasible.

If, for example, ample research evidence existed with respect to the science of nursing in its entirety, and if the definition of nursing published in the American Nurses Association's *Nursing: A Social Policy Statement* (1980) was unanimously endorsed, then the human response systems could provide a viable and engaging means of organizing a nursing curriculum. Nursing courses could be sequenced following each of the human response systems beginning with the physical response system and ending with the cultural response system. Or, courses could be sequenced following patterns of developmental theories in which age would become the primary organizer surrounded by appropriate age-related concepts and theories that would be accrued within each human response system. Similarly, other organizing themes such as the health-illness continuum could also provide a vehicle for organizing and delineating content using either a system-by-system or a cross-sectional approach to explicate each of the human response systems.

The utilization of human response systems as the major curricular focus not only allows for the application of nursing knowledge based upon research-derived evidence, but also clearly defines the second prototype, in which human responses precede health problems, as the most pertinent option for nurses to use while ministering their services to clients. The human response systems allow nurses to tend to all aspects of their clients' total life experiences—whether involving developmental life changes, acute or chronic health deviations, or cultural and environmental life stressors. Since human response systems represent and reflect individual experiences, nurses can focus on and individualize the care being provided. The relationship between physician and nurse becomes mutually cooperative when the physician cares for and treats the health problem(s) while the nurse assists his or her clients to either adapt or re-pattern their human responses and behaviors from detrimental to productive modes of function.

In this model, nursing interventions would result from research and reflect the independent judgment and decision-making ability of the professional nurse. While this curricular structure is perhaps premature, it is nonetheless an exciting example of the elasticity with which the model can be used.

A NURSING CURRICULUM BASED ON "NURSING THEORY AS A MODEL"

Conceptual frameworks using a published nursing theory provide another alternative on which nurse educators can logically and systematically structure a curriculum. Using this method allows students an opportunity to be exposed to at least one of the major theoretical positions currently being espoused by a theoretical leader of the profession. The decision to adopt a single nursing theory also provides an opportunity to test the extent to which the theory can be validly and reliably applied to the practice of nursing. However, using one nursing theory does limit the breadth of learning available when students are exposed to a variety of viewpoints. Contemporary nursing theories also contain specific content-based terms and definitions which suggest it would be necessary to adopt not only a specific framework but a distinctive language as well.

The Loomis/Wood Model, however, allows for superimposing any of the existing nursing theoretical frameworks with a minimum of effort. Indeed, work with the model suggests any of the nursing theories can be utilized within the Loomis/Wood Model framework without usually altering or changing the terminology associated with two of the three dimensions of the model. Thus, should a faculty decide to change the nursing theoretical context of a given curriculum at a future date, such changes could be easily accomplished without destroying the basic structure. Most nursing theories, when used as the organizing principle(s) for a curriculum, function along the third dimensions of the Loomis/Wood Model. Others could be integrated by incorporating concepts of the theory along either the Health Problem or Human Response axis of the model. This dimension of the model is concerned with the unique aspects of clinical decision making and includes the five stages of data collection, diagnosis, planning, treatment, and evaluation. Specific vocabularies associated with each of the nursing theories can be integrated into this dimension of the Loomis/Wood Model.

If, for example, a faculty would decide to utilize Roger's (1970, 1981) theory of Unitary Man, the data collection process would address such phenomena as patients' energy fields, patterns, and organization, all within the principles of helicy, resonancy, and complementarity fitting along the Human Response axis. The actual and potential health problems that are affected or included in the situation remain remarkably unchanged while the uniqueness of the nursing theory involved lies imbedded in the cubes in the model matrix and in clinical decision-making processes. Similarly, should a faculty prefer to utilize the theory of Roy (1984), the assessment of involved internal or external cognators, regulators, focal contextual stimuli, and so forth can be easily viewed within the human response system and clinical decision-making portions of the model. Thus, any one of the existing nursing theories can be easily integrated into the model without compromising its integrity. Further, should a change from one nursing theory to another be desired at a later time, it can be made easily and simply by altering the terms and definitions used to represent and operationalize various components of the model.

The specific prototype selected for use with a given nursing theory might depend on the particular concepts and processes contained within it. For example, the prototype in which health problems interact with human responses would seem appropriate for many of the nursing theories, including those of Rogers (1970, 1981), Orem (1985), Watson (1988), and others, while health problems preceding human responses might be more reflective of the theories postulated by Orlando (1961, 1972, 1987) and Peplau (1952, 1962). Content could be further organized according to particular strands or threads of a theory or by using the clinical decision-making processes associated with assessment and data collection, diagnosis, planning, treatment, and evaluation. Language specific to the nursing theory selected would be incorporated throughout the nursing courses and would provide the means by which nursing care would be identified and defined, and interventions structured.

CONCLUSION

This chapter suggests the Loomis/Wood Model of clinical nursing provides nurse educators with a viable alternative to existing options used as theoretical, conceptual, or organizing frameworks for structuring and organizing nursing content. The ability of the model to articulate easily and effectively with medically dominated material, the emerging knowledge relevant to caring for phenomena associated with one or more of the human response systems, or nursing theory, present some illustrations of its flexibility. In addition, the model can serve as a framework for either undergraduate or graduate level programs, and for those schools offering both types of educational programming—the model allows for effortless articulation between both.

It should be noted, however, that the model is not without its critics and criticism. Critics of the model express concerns with regard to what they perceive is an absence of attention focusing on the preventive aspects of nursing, particularly those areas that emphasize the nurse's role in health promotion related activities. Another area of concern relates to what some faculty perceive as a failure of the model to sufficiently address the domain of family nursing. It is difficult to determine whether or not these criticisms are sufficient to negate the overall structure and usefulness of the theory; however, they need to be heard and carefully considered.

It would seem likely that the concerns regarding the absence of focus on preventive measures could be explicated within the definition and parameters associated with the dimension labeled "potential health problems." Likewise, since one of the human response systems is delineated specifically as "family," it would seem possible for family-oriented content to be incorporated within the dimension designated as human response systems, or to use family as the domain for the entire model.

Finally, the recent emphasis and summons by nursing's educational leadership for a major curriculum revolution cannot be disregarded or overlooked (National League for Nursing, 1987). The need to prepare future students for a continually evolving and changing practice arena in a cost effective manner is being reiterated with increasing frequency by faculty and administrators alike. There is a need to develop innovative models of curriculum design that protects the paradigm of the profession relative to theory and practice. The move to surrender the legacy and dominance of behavioral objectives in favor of a more meaningful and socially responsive program of instruction is another dimension of the current mandate to revolutionize nursing school curricula. It should be noted, however, that most of the rhetoric concerning the need to revolutionize nursing curricula is targeted toward content and pedagogical changes rather than structural or framework oriented changes (Bevis & Watson, 1989). The Loomis/Wood Model is adaptable to changing content along three distinct dimensions. Therefore, faculties using this model can direct and maximize their efforts toward incorporating relevant content into the curriculum rather than spending an inordinate amount of time attempting to identify, agree upon, and then operationalize a specific narrowly defined theoretical, conceptual, or other organizing framework.

The Loomis/Wood Model is adaptable to the proposed curricular revolution because of its ability to accommodate to a wide variety of content and conceptual issues. It would seem probable that if faculties could adopt a stable organizing curricular framework like the Loomis/Wood Model, they could better utilize their time and effort in being more responsive to changing content, technology, and modes of practice. Perhaps the time saved from dealing with conceptual issues related to curricular structure could be redirected toward elucidating and responding to those content areas demanding a humanistic and artistic approach to care and caring in a variety of personal, professional, and global environments.

CASE STUDY ILLUSTRATION: THE LOOMIS/WOOD MODEL IN ONE SCHOOL'S CURRICULUM DESIGN

The baccalaureate degree nursing program at the University of Wisconsin-Eau Claire (UWEC) was first established in 1965. Since then, the nursing program has experienced continued growth and progress. In addition to the basic baccalaureate degree program, there is a satellite baccalaureate program established in cooperation with St. Joseph's Hospital in Marshfield, a separate educational track for registered nurses, a registered nurse to master's degree educational track, and a master's degree program allowing students the option to major in either Adult Health Nursing or in Family Health Nursing.

The concept and practice of change, as this brief description suggests, is a fact of life at the University of Wisconsin-Eau Claire. This level of change cannot be sustained without an innovative, flexible, and progressive curricular organizing framework. Curriculum revision at the institution has been continuous, with intermittent periodic burst of more major activity. The most recent major curricular revision occurred in 1983 when the nursing faculty revised its curriculum using an integrated conceptual approach to present nursing theory and knowledge as well as relevant interdisciplinary knowledge. The work of the faculty resulted in an organizing framework (Figure 2) based on developmental processes, the metaparadigm of the discipline of nursing, and the clinical nursing model developed by Loomis and Wood (1983). The purpose of this case study is to describe how these components combine to guide the theoretical and clinical development and teaching of clinical components of each of the various curricula.

PHILOSOPHY OF THE UWEC SCHOOL OF NURSING

A unique aspect of the UWEC School of Nursing is that both the undergraduate and graduate programs as well as their associated tracks operate from one school of nursing philosophy and one organizing curricular framework. Such an approach allows curriculum development to proceed in a logical and systematic fashion with the basic foundation providing support across courses, departments, and programs.

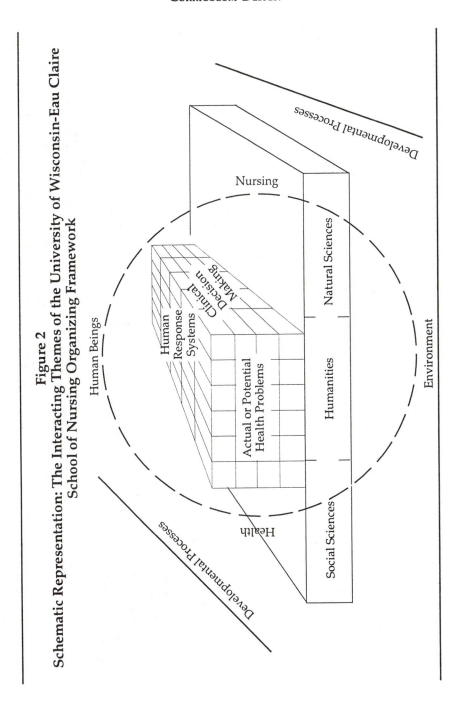

Figure 2
Schematic Representation: The Interacting Themes of the University of Wisconsin-Eau Claire
School of Nursing Organizing Framework

The school of nursing philosophy is consistent with the mission of the university, and the faculty believes in the value of a liberal education as the foundation for both pre-professional and professional programs.

The philosophy also incorporates the faculty's beliefs regarding the four phenomena of the discipline's predominant paradigm: nursing, human beings, environment, and health. An organizing framework and glossary of terms offer more precise definitions and show interrelationships among these terms, developmental processes, and the Loomis/Wood Model.

The organizing framework provides direction for the selection and sequencing of content in all of the educational programs. The three components, the phenomena of the discipline, developmental processes, and the Loomis/Wood Model, each have a specific function in the framework.

The *Loomis/Wood Model* provides for the systematic study of relationships among actual and potential health problems, human responses, and clinical decision making (see Figure 1). The model proposes four categories for actual or potential health problems. Six human response systems are identified governing how individuals respond to health problems. The third dimension of the model describes the clinical decision-making process. This constitutes application of the nursing process and effectively guides clinical learning experiences for students in both programs.

Phenomena of the discipline serves as one parameter for the selection of specific theories and concepts to be included in the programs. Some salient beliefs include: (1) Human beings are multifaceted, develop progressively, and respond to actual and potential health problems. (2) Clients are individuals, but families, groups, and communities as clients also reflect these qualities. (3) The environment comprises multiple external factors which change, develop, and interact with each other and with human beings.

Health is an individually defined state which reflects human responses to developmental life changes, acute and chronic health deviations, and environmental factors. This state changes in human beings with changes in responses to actual and potential health problems. Nursing is a theory-based professional discipline which uses clinical decision making to diagnose and treat human responses to actual and potential health problems. Nursing research relates theories and concepts to practice. Nursing is a blend of scientific and affective characteristics and is practiced in a variety of roles and settings. Nurses collaborate with clients and their supportive persons, and with other health care providers.

Subconcepts of the phenomena such as leadership, decision making, coping, and research have been identified by graduate and undergraduate faculties. Prerequisite courses are chosen to ensure that students are prepared to study the concepts and subconcepts, and to ensure intellectual skills which are used throughout in nursing courses.

Developmental processes provide the logic for sequencing content within courses and courses within programs. Theoretical content precedes application of that content. Undergraduate clinical courses sequence content using human development from conception through older adulthood. Theoretical content using developmental theory in the graduate program focuses on the developmental processes of adulthood and families in a variety of settings.

OPERATIONALIZING THE CONCEPTUAL FRAMEWORK: UNDERGRADUATE CURRICULUM

A strong theoretical base in the natural and social sciences is provided students in the pre-professional curriculum. Humanities courses are also incorporated throughout the program of study. Nursing courses build on content from prerequisite course work and assist students to integrate knowledge from the sciences and humanities with contemporary professional knowledge.

Theoretical nursing courses provide scientific knowledge about theories and concepts relevant to the four phenomena of nursing. The student uses the three components of the Loomis/Wood Model in determining diagnoses and treatments for human responses to actual and potential health problems. This model is used primarily in the clinical courses in the undergraduate curriculum. It also is an integral part of the theory and practicum courses in the graduate curriculum.

Three of the five undergraduate clinical courses focus specifically on the developmental stages of human beings: conception through adolescence, young adult to midlife, and midlife through older adulthood. Table 1 identifies the sequencing and content focus of each of the required nursing courses.

Table 1
Required Nursing Courses

Course	Theory (T) Clinical (C)	Content Focus
N210 Health Dimensions	T (Open to all majors)	Health concepts, personal health concerns and responsibilities, health care services
N215 Professional Dimensions of Nursing	T	Nursing history, education, research, theories, and practice.
N225/226* Practice Dimensions of Nursing	C	Introduces clinical decision making (emphasis on individuals across the lifespan). Focus on interpersonal skills, health assessment, teaching, and selected nursing skills. CDM* focus data collection and assessment. Application of N210, 215 content.
N310 Societal Dimensions of Nursing	T	Family, group, and community theories. Ethical decision making models. Interrelationships between human responses and environment.
N315 & N320 Scientific Dimensions of Nursing I and II	T	Pathophysiologic and psychopathologic processes across the lifespan. Nutritional and pharmacologic therapy.
N325 Nursing Conception through Adolescence	C	CDM focus on data analysis and nursing diagnosis. Individuals as clients. Application of N225, N310, N315 content.

Course	Type	Description
N355 Nursing: Young Adult to Midlife	C	CDM focus on outcome, criteria and nursing treatments. Individuals and families as clients. Application of N325, N320 content.
N415 Management Dimensions of Nursing	T	Organizational behavior, leadership and management theory. Health care system and societal influences.
N425/426* Nursing Midlife through Older Adulthood	C	CDM focus on evaluation and revision. Individuals, families, and groups as clients. Application of N355 content.
N455/456* Transitions to Professional Practice	C	Integration of leadership and management skills with CDM. Diverse clinical settings and client populations, including the community as a client. Application of N425, N415 content.
N475 Professional Seminar	T	Contemporary issues affecting nursing. Research issues and process.

*Indicates corresponding course in RN/BSN program.
CDM = clinical decison making

OPERATIONALIZING THE CONCEPTUAL FRAMEWORK: FACULTY DEVELOPMENT AND EXPERIENCES

Transition to a conceptually based nursing curriculum required faculty development. During the process of revision, three faculty attended an international nurse-theorists' conference. Other faculty attended a conference on designing conceptually based and integrated nursing curricula led by Gertrude Torres. These faculty returned with enthusiasm and commitment as well as basic information to share with other faculty. This set the stage for knowledge and attitude shifts required to make significant curricular changes.

After reviewing the school's philosophy, faculty considered various nursing and related theories in order to develop a conceptual framework. It was at this time, in 1983, that the Loomis and Wood article was published. This model, when considered with developmental theories and the phenomena of the discipline, offered enough specificity to guide curriculum development. It also was general and flexible enough to guide planning efforts in specific courses. The Loomis/Wood Model identified nursing concerns and processes in a way which permitted use of a variety of nursing and related theories, rather than designing a curriculum based on a particular nursing theory. This was believed to be more desirable both because of the faculty's philosophy of nursing and education, and because of the fluid state of nursing theory development.

Upon making the decision to use the clinical model, Maxine Loomis was invited to discuss the model with faculty and to address faculty questions and concerns. Two faculty inservices and several consultation sessions were provided by Dr. Loomis. Numerous faculty discussions preceded and followed consultation with Dr. Loomis. Because the model had not been operationalized in an educational setting, faculty needed to come to consensus about the operationalization process. Two major areas of concern were the extent to which the model would direct content selection and organization and how the clinical decision-making process would be used in the clinical courses. Faculty achieved sufficient agreement to move ahead with development of the curriculum. However, these two major issues continue to be topics of active discussion.

Changes within the courses based on student and faculty evaluations have occurred over the last six years. However, only one major curriculum revision has been made. Originally N315 and N320 Scientific Dimensions of Nursing (see Table 1) was a single five-credit course. This proved to be both an insufficient amount of time to cover the required material and an overwhelming academic challenge for students. This content is now offered as two three-credit courses.

Because the 1985 National League for Nursing (NLN) accreditation visit occurred as one curriculum was ending and another starting, a progress report on the revised curriculum was submitted to the NLN in 1989. Results of the NLN review were gratifying. The NLN Board of Review granted continuing accreditation, noting that substantial progress had been made in meeting previous Board recommendations. The only curricular recommendation concerned the need for clarification of some general education prerequisite courses. Overall, the board of review congratulated the school of nursing in its continued efforts to offer a quality nursing education program.

While changes both positive and negative have been noted in alumni and employer perceptions of the quality of the undergraduate education and preparation of graduates, overall impressions of both groups remain positive. One difficulty of comparing evaluations of current graduates is the fact that the evaluation instrument was designed using the previous curricular objectives. A comparison of the previous and the revised curriculum using the same instrument was felt to be necessary initially. However, new instruments using objectives of the revised curriculum will not be used to obtain data specifically about this curriculum.

For the three graduating classes, the NCLEX pass rate has been higher than the national pass rate and higher than or equivalent to the Wisconsin rate. However, UWEC has traditionally had a pass rate of 95 percent or better. Faculty are concerned that we maintain our norm rather than the national or state norm. Efforts are underway to identify specific ways to improve teaching methods and facilitate student learning. So far, a key area of concern is the identification of better ways to help students transfer information from the theoretical courses to clinical practice.

As noted previously, an issue which faculty have needed to address concerns the teaching of the clinical decision-making process. While the Loomis/Wood Model clearly identifies *what* is to be taught, it does not address *how* it should be taught. Faculty recently decided that clinical decision-making (CDM) should be taught in a sequential way, with subsequent clinical courses building on skills emphasized in previous courses. Faculty and students would always be aware of the entire CDM process, but focus and emphasis in student learning activities would be on specifically identified CDM components.

Emphasis of some of the components of the clinical decision-making process within specific courses can be found in Table 1. Future evaluation will need to address whether or not students are more proficient in clinical decision making when the process is taught in this manner.

While there are faculty who still prefer the previous curriculum, the majority of faculty agree that the revised curriculum is superior. The focus is on nursing theory and practice. The consistency of language and speech across the curriculum is beneficial to students. Students have the opportunity to learn many different views and theories of nursing within a unified conceptual framework. Thus, the ambiguities of nursing can be discussed while maintaining the integrity of the curriculum.

An unanticipated benefit of using the Loomis/Wood Model as part of the conceptual framework has been that one of the acute care agencies associated with the school of nursing has also adopted the model to guide clinical nursing practice. Students who have a clinical experience in this agency have the opportunity to work in a philosophically consistent setting.

FUTURE CONSIDERATIONS

Course content is a critical element in the curricular design and requires ongoing systematic monitoring to ensure the integrity of the curricula. The school of nursing evaluation plan is currently being assessed and refined to ensure that essential evaluation data is documented in a way which uses faculty time efficiently. Content and concept mapping are ongoing to provide direction in continuing efforts to increase internal consistency throughout the curriculum.

Some questions remain to be answered by faculty. Should elective courses be guided by the existing conceptual framework, or should they be an opportunity for faculty and students to explore other conceptual frameworks? How much opportunity to work with specific nursing theories should be incorporated at the undergraduate level? What is the best way for faculty to maintain expertise and identity in a clinical practice area while teaching in an integrated curriculum?

A shared philosophy and organizing framework have provided continuity across undergraduate and graduate programs and have facilitated developments such as an RN/MSN option. This option provides the opportunity for qualifying registered nurses to pursue a bachelor of science in nursing degree and a master of science in nursing degree in an accelerated program of study. This and other innovative options such as an accelerated baccalaureate degree are possible to implement because the organizing framework provides curricular guidelines in a flexible manner. Furthermore, the unifying organizing framework serves to maintain the integrity of both the undergraduate and graduate degrees.

REFERENCES

American Nurses' Association (1980). *Nursing: A social policy statement.* Kansas City, MO: Author.

Bevis, E. O. (1982). *Curriculum building in nursing: A process* (3rd ed.). St. Louis: C. V. Mosby.

Bevis, E. O. (1989). *Curriculum building in nursing: A process* (3rd ed.). New York: National League for Nursing.

Bevis, E. O., & Watson, J. (1989). *Toward a caring curriculum: A new pedagogy for nursing.* New York: National League for Nursing.

Chater, S. S. (1975). A conceptual framework for curriculum development. *Nursing Outlook, 23,* 428–433.

Goldmark, J. (1923). *Nursing and nursing education in the United States.* New York: Macmillan.

Kelly, L. Y. (1985). *Dimensions of professional nursing* (5th ed.). New York: Macmillan.

Loomis, M., & Wood, D. (1983). Cure: The potential outcome of nursing. *Image: The Journal of Nursing Scholarship, 15,* 4–7.

National League for Nursing. (1985). *Policies and procedures of accreditation for programs in nursing education.* New York: Author.

National League for Nursing. (1987). *Curriculum revolution: Mandate for change.* New York: Author.

Orem, D. E. (1985). *Nursing—Concepts of practice* (3rd ed.). New York: McGraw-Hill

Orlando, I. J. (1961). *The dynamic nurse-patient relationship.* New York: Putnam's Sons.

Orlando, I. J. (1972). *The discipline and teaching of nursing process.* New York: Putnam's Sons.

Orlando, I. J. (1987). Nursing in the twenty-first century: Alternate paths. *Journal of Advanced Nursing, 12*(4), 405–412.

Peplau, H. E. (1952). *Interpersonal relations in nursing.* New York: Putnam's Sons.

Peplau, H. E. (1962). Interpersonal techniques: The crux of psychiatric nursing. *The American Journal of Nursing, 62*(6), 50–54.

Rogers, M. E. (1970). *An introduction to the theoretical basis of nursing.* Philadelphia: Davis.

Rogers, M. E. (1981). A science of unitary man: A paradigm for nursing. In G. E. Laskar (Ed.), *Applied systems and cybernetics.* New York: Pergamon.

Roy, C. (1984). *Introduction to nursing: An adaptation model.* Englewood Cliffs, NJ: Prentice-Hall.

Santora, D. (1980). *Conceptual frameworks used in baccalaureate and master's degree curricula.* New York: National League for Nursing.

Torres, G., & Stanton, M. (1982). *Curriculum process in nursing: A guide to curriculum development.* Englewood Cliffs, NJ: Prentice-Hall.

Watson, J. (1988). *Nursing: Human science and human care.* New York: National League for Nursing.

3

Application and Utilization of the Loomis/Wood Model as the Conceptual Framework for the Conduct of Nursing Research

Joan Stehle Werner

*F*or over three decades, nurses have been engaged increasingly in the conduct of research. As a result, the publication and presentation of nursing research has grown dramatically. This expansion of research productivity is evidenced in the evolution of the number of nursing research journals from one in 1952 to eight nursing journals with either "research," "inquiry," "scholarship," or "science" in their titles in 1990. This increase represents an expotential rise in the number of published nursing research reports in the past 38 years, not withstanding the numerous research reports included in journals specific to certain clinical specialties, and other nursing journals. While the commitment and dedication of the profession and discipline of nursing to research is beyond question, what is not yet as clear is what the focus of nursing research should be. This issue has been debated for as long as nurses have been engaged in research (see, for example, Gortner, 1990; Schultz & Meleis, 1988; Webster, Jacox, & Baldwin, 1981).

The issue of the focus of nursing research is deeply entwined with a related issue, that of what nursing is. What nursing is has also been

49

a topic of momentous analysis and debate for over three decades. The definition of nursing as the meeting of intrapersonal needs of the patient (Henderson, 1964, 1966) has taken a long and convoluted pathway to several current conceptions of nursing, for example, nursing conceptualized as human caring (Watson, 1988), with no uncontended conclusion visible in the near future. Until the question of what nursing is is resolved, nurse researchers will not have a clear direction as to the central focus for nursing research. Contrarily, perhaps the nursing inquiry being accomplished at present will facilitate or lead nursing to a clearer demarcation of its knowledge domain.

In the interim, until nursing converges on an acceptable definition and resulting domain of phenomena for study, the discipline is still in need of demarcations to guide its areas of research concentration. One purpose of this chapter is to explain how the Loomis/Wood Model can be used to guide the sphere of nursing research content. Examples of the utility of the model in directing selection of nursing research substance will be given.

A second purpose of this chapter is to describe the versatility of the Loomis/Wood Model in serving as a model for research stemming from competing paradigms for the conduct of research. As a content framework, the model is useful with the humanist/interpretive research paradigm as well as with the more traditional hypothetico/deductive or positivist/empiricist paradigm of research strategies (Woods & Catanzaro, 1988). Illustrations of the use of the model in research stemming from differing paradigms will also be described.

DOMAIN OF THE LOOMIS/WOOD MODEL

The usefulness of the Loomis/Wood Model as a blueprint for nursing research rests on the scope or domain of the phenomena of concern which it encompasses. While there is yet no firm concurrence on what nursing is, the Loomis/Wood Model was developed to portray nursing phenomena as conceptualized in the American Nurses' Association's (ANA, 1980) *Nursing: A social policy statement.* Although this definition of nursing has achieved widespread support in nursing, its acclaim is far from unanimous.

The scope of the phenomena depicted in the model, therefore, flows from the ANA definition of nursing as "the diagnosis and treatment of human responses to actual or potential health problems" (ANA, 1980, p. 9). According to Dubin (1978), when analyzed, this definition implies a set of linear "sequential" relationships in which a health problem (actual or potential) precedes human responses. The nurse then collects data regarding diagnoses and treats these human responses, whereby cure of the actual or potential health problem can be achieved. In developing their model, Loomis and Wood (1983) made the assumption that interactions between health problems, human responses, nursing, and cure were rarely simply linear, because "any factor in the equation can affect any other" (p. 4). Therefore, their model was developed as a multivariate cube in which all human response systems interact with all actual or potential health problems and to which nursing clinical decision making can be applied, yielding an even more intricate cubical multivariate framework (see Chapter 1 for a more detailed explanation of the Loomis/ Wood Model).

One major assumption captured by the Loomis/Wood Model, then, is that phenomena of concern to nursing are multivariate in nature. This central assumption coincides clearly with nursing's current and serious regard for the complexity of human experiences.

The scope of the Loomis/Wood Model and its utility in delimiting content for nursing research can be further appreciated by recounting the phenomena which form the three axes of the cube. Two of these axes are content axes, while the third is a process axis. The vertical axis depicted in Figure 1 is one of the content axes and represents Actual or Potential Health Problems which are categorized as: (a) developmental life changes, (b) acute health deviations, (c) chronic health deviations, or (d) culturally and environmentally induced stressors. The horizontal content axis encompasses Human Response Systems including: (a) physical, (b) emotional, (c) cognitive, (d) family, (e) social, and (f) cultural. The remaining process axis provides for nursing as part of the model and is labeled Clinical Decision Making. According to Loomis and Wood (1983), "Clinical decision making as proposed in this model follows the familiar problem-solving steps of the nursing process" (p. 4) (see Figure 1). Flaskerud and Halloran (1980) argue that the concept of nursing should be contained in a theory if it is to be labeled uniquely a nursing theory. By the same token, the Loomis/Wood Model can be considered a nursing conceptual framework since it includes clinical decision making or the nursing process.

The domain of phenomena bounded by the model also corre-

Figure 1
Model for the Study of Clinical Nursing

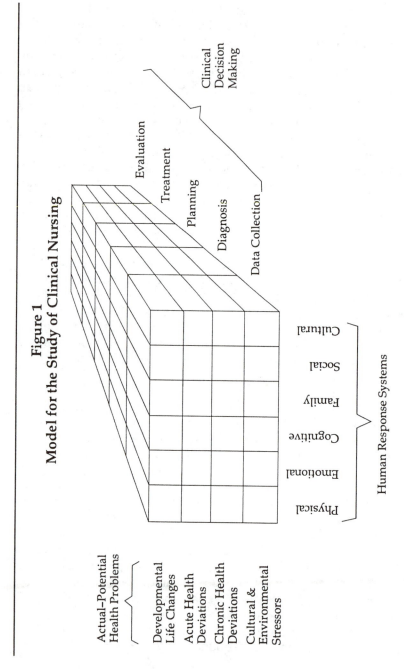

From "Cure: The Potential Outcome of Nursing Care," by M. Loomis and D. Wood, *Image 15*, p. 4. Reprinted by permission.

sponds fittingly with the four major concepts analyzed by Fawcett (1984) to constitute the metaparadigm of nursing. These summative concepts, presumably the central themes for nursing research, include: Human Being, Health, Environment, and Nursing. As constructs, human being and health are evidenced in the model by the inclusion of the perpendicular and horizontal axes, Actual or Potential Health Problems and Human Responses, which are central to the interaction of people with health and or health concerns. Environment, while not specifically detailed in the cubicular schema of the model, is implied to pervade the phenomena in the model since all actual or potential health problems as well as all human responses occur in interaction with a certain environment or environments. In addition, environment is also inferred to subsume the entire framework since nursing clinical decision making is also conducted within an environment which may have great bearing on the outcome of the nurse-client process (see Figure 2). Nursing as a major construct is obviously and straightforwardly represented by the Clinical Decision-Making process axis. It is also implied as a boundary for the core of the model since, by definition, nurses are the professionals most centrally involved with the intersection of human beings, their health, health problems, and their related human responses (ANA, 1980). Figure 2 also signifies the importance of the social sciences, humanities, and natural sciences to nursing.

The scope of the model, therefore, is broad yet specific to nursing. Because of this flexible nature, the Loomis/Wood Model is a fitting framework to guide nursing research whether the investigation is considerable in scope or explicitly precise in nature. For example, it is extensive enough to allow for study of factors such as cultural stressors affecting human beings which may or may not ultimately have bearing on health. It is elaborate enough to permit investigation of the subjective reality of people experiencing life changes. It is broad enough to guide a researcher to the examination of person-environment fit.

Yet, in addition to the model's liberal scope, it is also tolerant and supportive of inquiry regarding, for example, specific cognitions resulting from a health problem, particular physiological processes associated with acute illness, or individual patterns of human responses which precede chronic conditions. Moreover, the model's inclusion of the clinical decision-making process underscores the need for research regarding the operations through which effective nursing can be carried out. The Loomis/Wood Model, then, is an apt

Figure 2

Nursing's Meta Paradigm Concepts as Boundaries for the Domain of the Loomis/Wood Model

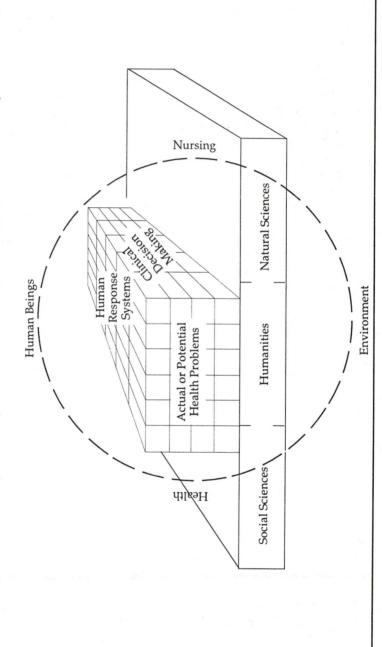

framework for application and utilization in the conduct of nursing research and a worthy guide to the currently acceptable domain of phenomena for nursing inquiry.

USES OF THE MODEL AS A FRAMEWORK FOR NURSING RESEARCH

In the preceding portion of this chapter, the usefulness of the Loomis/ Wood Model as a guide for nursing research was advocated. This section provides a more detailed look at the flexibility of the model as a framework for nursing research.

The Loomis/Wood Model is a conceptual framework. As such, it provides abstract concepts which separately or in concert can direct or guide selection of content for nursing research. While the model in its entirety depicts a multivariate focus, the model can also be used to suggest research focusing on subconcepts subsumed within each of the three axes or on transactions formed through the interaction of subconcepts from two of the three axes, or with all three axes.

RESEARCH WITHIN AXES OF THE MODEL

Using the Loomis/Wood Model as a content guide could conceivably lead to the study of phenomena within any of the three axes. Nurse researchers may have research questions or problems which pertain to actual or potential health problems themselves. Or, they might choose to investigate topics fitting within either of the two remaining axes. Each of the subconcepts within any of the axes could provide numerous topics for nursing research.

Actual or Potential Health Problems

According to Loomis and Wood (1983), actual or potential health problems, the first dimension of the model, may include developmental life changes, acute health deviations, chronic health deviations, or culturally or environmentally induced stressors, all worthy of extended investigation. Loomis and Wood note that without the presence of at least one of these four factors, there exists no actual or potential health problem.

Developmental life changes are "transitional processes related to growth, maturation or changes in life related to aging" (UWEC Faculty, 1984, p. 2.913). According to Loomis and Wood (1983), this category of actual or potential health problems includes transitions or events such as puberty, marriage, pregnancy, divorce, retirement, and similar episodes. Each life event can *signify* or precipitate actual or potential health problems. Acute health deviations are defined as "time limited departures from normal functioning," while chronic health deviations are defined as "long-term departures from normal functioning" (UWEC Faculty, 1984, p. 2.913). Loomis and Wood's (1983) examples of acute health deviations include injuries, diseases, and invasive organisms. Chronic health deviations are described as usually requiring "changes in lifestyle" (p. 6). Examples include diabetes and chronic respiratory disease.

Cultural/environmental stressors are "external forces that require a change or modification in functioning" (UWEC Faculty, 1984, p. 2.913). Such forces may be economic, legal, organizational, political, or religious in nature. Economic conditions, such as unemployment, as well as certain norms or customs and other stressors, are considered culturally or environmentally induced.

Research could focus solely within any of the broad concepts just described. Within the Actual or Potential Health Problem axis, for example, investigations could focus on the developmental life changes associated with the transition to being a step-parent. The actual or potential health problems associated with this particular developmental life change could be examined and specified, thereby eliciting a more thorough classification of actual or potential health problems for this particular phase. Studies of this nature could yield a compendium of subconcepts of actual or potential health problems for each category specified along the vertical content axis of the model. Results of these studies could then be useful in further investigations of the human responses to each subcategory of actual or potential health problems. Once these studies were completed, researchers could include aspects of the clinical decision-making process, yielding related nursing diagnoses, and specifying the most effective and efficient treatments for diagnoses.

Case example.   An example of the type of research specified above was included as part of a larger study conducted at the University of Wisconsin-Eau Claire by Silko (1985). The purposes of Silko's overall descriptive and correlational cross-sectional study were to identify age-related actual and potential health problems and human responses of employed adult women in the areas of health, education, family, career, and self. Two of the five research questions for this study were specifically aimed at discerning actual and/or potential health problems of the women. These questions included:

1. Do three age-related groups of employed adult women differ in what they identify as their concerns related to actual or potential health problems?
2. What association, if any, exists between selected cultural/environmental factors and the actual and potential health problem concerns of employed adult women?

A convenience sample of 200 women was randomly selected from employees of two institutions, one health care and one higher education, in a small Midwestern city. Data were collected by means of a questionnaire developed by the investigator and mailed to the women's homes. There was a 73 percent response rate ($n = 46$). The majority of women were in the young adult group, between ages 18 and 45, employed by a hospital, working full-time, earning between $20,000 and $40,000 per year, had completed some schooling after high school, were married, and had children. The middle-adult group (46–55 years) comprised 16 percent of the sample ($n = 24$), while older adult women numbered 21 (14%).

As defined by the University of Wisconsin-Eau Claire nursing faculty (1984), the conceptual definitions used for this study included: (1) *Cultural/Environmental factors:* external forces that require a change or modification in functioning; (2) *Actual health problem:* instability or decline in health status related to developmental life changes, acute or chronic health deviations, or cultural/environmental stressors; (c) *Potential health problem:* health status characterized by risk factors which could lead to actual health problems; (d) *Concern:* a potential health problem; and (e) *Developmental life changes:* transitional processes related to growth, maturation, or changes in life related to aging.

Findings indicated that women in this study expressed concerns related to actual or potential health problems in several areas including career/job, health status, financial status, educational status, self, marital relationship, and relationship with children and relationship with parents. Highest levels of concerns for women in the youngest group related to career/job, educational status, and relationships with children. The middle age group was mostly concerned about their career/job, health status, and relationships with children, while the older women were the most concerned about self, financial status, and relationship with spouse.

The mean frequency of actual or potential health-related concerns reported by young adult women was 3.1, for the middle adult group it was 3.3, while the mean was 2.4 for the older group of women. Regarding health concerns, the women of the youngest age group had the highest level of concern about their health status. As a whole, the majority of women reported having experienced only one or two major health problems at the time of the survey. The most frequently experienced health problems indicated by each of the groups were menstrual problems for the younger adult women, bladder or vaginal infections for the middle-aged women, and menstrual problems, bladder infections, or accidental injuries for the oldest group of women. Although the women of all the groups reported a moderately high level of concern, the groups did not differ significantly in their reported levels of concern.

Regarding associations between cultural/environmental factors and actual or potential health problems, significant correlations were found in the following areas: (1) between level of concern regarding relationships with children and both the number of hours worked per week and the number of roles performed; (2) between level of educational achievement and level of expressed satisfaction with career, educational status, and self; (3) between the number of roles regularly performed by the women and their self-satisfaction; and (4) between level of satisfaction with marital status and household yearly income.

Results of this study demonstrate that the Loomis/Wood Model is useful in organizing studies related to nursing, particularly those which further identify concerns related to actual or potential health problems. This particular study provides information regarding the major concerns of adult women, their identified actual or potential health problems, and related factors, within one axis of the model.

Human Response System Axis

The Loomis/Wood Model can also be useful in guiding research regarding human responses. The ability to study specific human responses or human response systems within this framework is a particularly unique and attractive feature of the model. According to the University of Wisconsin-Eau Claire faculty (1984), human responses are defined as "behaviors that can be described as scientifically explained" (p. 2.913).

The human response systems make up the second, or horizontal, axis of the model (see Figure 1). This dimension of the model is central to the definition of nursing forwarded by the American Nurses' Association (1980). Loomis and Wood (1983) propose there are six human response systems through which a person responds to actual or potential health problems: (1) Physical—"of or pertaining to material things, natural sciences of the body"; (2) Emotional—"of or pertaining to affective aspect of consciousness, a state of feeling"; (3) Cognitive—"of or pertaining to knowledge, perception, reason, intuition or thought"; (4) Family—"of or pertaining to responses reflecting participation with relatives and significant others"; (5) Social—"of or pertaining to relationships with informal and formal organizations within society"; and (6) Cultural (including spiritual)—"of or pertaining to normative behavior patterns, values and mores" (UWEC faculty, 1984, p. 2.913). The individual may respond to an actual or potential problem with responses in one or in a number of response systems.

While human responses usually are studied in relation to some actual or potential health problem, it is conceivable that investigators could study response patterns solely within the second axis. For example, in studying the human responses which are characteristic of anxiety, the stimulus or related threat, according to some scholars, may not be identified. Yet, the patterns of human responses can still be identified (Whitley, 1989). The seminal studies conducted and guided by Norris (1982) are excellent illustrations of this type of research yielding human response pattern indicators.

For instance, Anderson (1982) studied the concept of hunger by interviewing 16 nurses and interviewing and observing nine patients. Patient charts and anecdotal notes were also examined. She identified three categories of evidence denoting hunger, including: (1) behaviors, further categorized into preoccupation, increased activity, and emotional lability; (2) internal experiences, further subcategorized as gastrointestinal hypermotility, feelings related to emotional lability, and decreased energy; and (3) affect. Anderson went on to develop "the hunger continuum" (p. 203) which consisted of three phases: initial hunger, progression of hunger, and extreme and long duration hunger. She specified behavioral manifestations for each phase. These manifestations or human responses occurred most frequently in the physical, emotional, and cognitive human response systems. Through her study, Anderson identified unique patterns of human responses indicative of types of hunger. In this particular study, the specific underlying causes of hunger were not the focus of study, although they were discussed. Instead, the defining characteristics or manifestations of the concept *hunger* were determined through the investigation yielding a pattern of human responses which, when operationally assessed, can be used both to identify hunger and distinguish phases of a process involving this increasingly serious condition.

Other excellent examples of research involving the identification of the coalescence of human responses in discernible patterns are found within the growing research literature on nursing diagnoses (Johnson, 1989; Mahoney, 1989). The focus of these studies is on defining characteristics or manifestations of certain diagnoses. These manifestations all fit within one or more of the human response systems. It is the uniqueness of each set of interrelated responses that can be identified through research, yielding an identifiable phenomenon labeled diagnosis.

Research within the Human Response System axis can proceed from particular to general or from the phenomenon to the specific human responses. In the first instance, nurses may observe certain human responses occurring in related patterns which may suggest, and with further study may render, a new or as yet undescribed entity (see, for example, Smith's 1988 study of deterioration). In the second scenario, a known concept could be the focal point of an investigation in which distinctive traits or features are identified and operationally defined (see, for example, MacLean, 1989). This second method of examining the human responses that contribute to a conceptual pattern is illustrated in the following case example.

Case example.   Oleson (1984) studied the phenomenon of postsurgical fatigue. The purpose of her research was to identify and describe patterns of observable manifestations and subjective responses of postsurgical fatigue in a clinical setting. The Loomis/Woods Model for the study of clinical nursing provided the conceptual framework for the study, which employed a descriptive exploratory design.

The population for this study consisted of adult patients admitted to the general surgical unit of a community hospital for elective abdominal surgery. A convenience sample of ten females undergoing cholecystectomy and total abdominal hysterectomy was selected and a pilot-tested observation checklist and a self-rating scale were used to collect data. The participants were observed for manifestations of fatigue and asked to rate subjective responses of fatigue pre-operatively and during the first three consecutive postoperative days. According to Oleson (1984), "Recognizing that none of the categories of human response systems is independent or mutually exclusive, three were considered most relevant for this study. These three were the physical, emotional, and cognitive response systems" (p. 3) (see Figure 3).

Results of this study signified patterns of observed manifestations for three consecutive postoperative days. Most frequent human responses present in these patterns were: (1) needing assistance with daily living activities, (2) droopy eyelids, (3) slow and clumsy movements, (4) grimacing, (5) avoiding conversation, and (6) inability to listen or concentrate. Fewer observed manifestations were recorded each successive postoperative day. Patterns of self-reported subjective responses of fatigue included: weakness, exhaustion, lack of appetite, lack of interest, sleepiness, and pain.

These findings attest to the existence of postsurgical fatigue in this surgical sample and suggested the observable manifestations and subjective responses of postsurgical fatigue. As such, postsurgical fatigue was better conceptualized through this research. As a result of this type of research, nurses should be able to further clarify human response phenomena and devise, implement, and test nursing measures to predict or alleviate any negative responses associated with the phenomenon of postsurgical fatigue, and other salient phenomena, by first clearly describing their particular patterns of human responses.

Nursing Clinical Decision-Making Axis

Nursing research can also be conducted using Loomis and Wood's third axis, the Clinical Decision-Making process axis, as a guide. Investigations specific to this axis would focus on how nurses either do or ideally can carry out the nursing process in an effective and efficient manner.

While research solely regarding clinical decision making could be

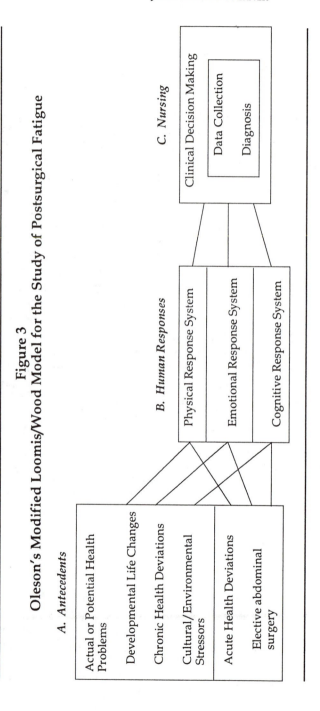

Figure 3
Oleson's Modified Loomis/Wood Model for the Study of Postsurgical Fatigue

done using the Loomis and Wood (1983) framework, the authors acknowledge that this specific framework would not be necessary to study this process. Numerous studies have been conducted regarding diagnostic reasoning, attention to cues in the diagnostic process, clinical judgment, planning, intervening, and evaluation. Ideally, studies of clinical decision making employing the Loomis and Wood framework would be specific to the human responses associated with actual or potential health problems.

Research Interrelating Axes of the Model

While it is feasible that investigations stemming exclusively from one of the three axes of the model could be implemented, the more likely scenario is one in which either two of the axes of the model are utilized, or studies employing portions of all three axes. At least 12 theses conducted at the University of Wisconsin-Eau Claire in the past seven years have converged on interrelations of selected dimensions of the Actual or Potential Health Problem axis together with aspects of the Human Response System axis, sometimes including the Clinical Decision-Making step of data collection or diagnosis (Gale-Swanson, 1986; Kafka, 1986; Kuznar, 1988; Oleson, 1984; Paremski, 1989; Rock, 1987; Schams, 1988; Silko, 1985; Smith, 1988; Sperstad, 1988; Vanderwalker, 1984; Woodruff, 1985). Several of these studies have yielded results which provide the groundwork for further delineation of nursing diagnoses or which suggest preliminary conclusions pointing to the need for further study of certain concepts and their unique patterns of human responses.

It is with the study of the interrelations of human responses with actual or potential health problems that this framework for research most closely coincides with the ANA (1980) definition of nursing. Future studies using interrelated axes of the model could contribute greatly to the knowledge base for nursing.

For example, the life-span developmental research methods espoused for nursing by Weekes and Rankin (1988) exemplify research pertaining to the combination of vertical and horizontal content axes of the Loomis/Wood Model. They support investigation within these two axes when they describe life-span research as that which examines "the nature of altered health status by surveying individual responses to illness in different age groups. These influences of age, time of measurement (period), and cohort on developmental change in response to varied health and illness conditions are of particular interest" (p. 380). This quote contains specific references not only to human responses, but also to combinations of developmental life changes with either acute or chronic health deviations. Inquiries focusing on transactions within the two content axes have also been conducted.

The previously mentioned study by Silko (1985), in its entirety, sought to ascertain human responses to developmental life change and actual and potential health problems of adult employed women. Oleson's (1984) study converged on patterns of human responses associated with the acute health deviation event of abdominal surgery. The following two case examples also illustrate the utility of the Loomis and Wood Model in guiding nursing research with interrelated aspects of the model.

Case examples.   In 1986, Kafka conducted thesis research investigating the concept of powerlessness among fathers involved with the birth experience either through cesarean birth or through vaginal delivery. For this study, fathering, or the experience of becoming the father of a new child, was viewed as a developmental life change, the first category of Actual or Potential Health Problems in the model. Fathering and type of delivery were conceptualized as potential health problems. The nursing diagnosis of powerlessness was conceptualized as inclusive of human responses in the social, cognitive, and emotional human response systems. It was the assumption of the study that the fathers' social, cognitive, and emotional responses to the birth experience could be assessed in order to establish knowledge regarding powerlessness, which could then assist nurses in preventing negative outcomes and encouraging positive outcomes for fathers in either type of birth experience. Kafka compared human responses between the two groups of fathers, those whose wives experienced cesarean birth and those who had vaginal deliveries.

The study design was descriptive using a convenience sample. Fifty fathers comprised the sample for the study with 25 fathers whose spouses had vaginal deliveries and 25 fathers whose wives had cesarean deliveries within a two- to three-month period of time. A written questionnaire was mailed to each father one week following delivery. Both the Loomis/Wood Model and the concept of powerlessness provided the basis for selecting items used in constructing the questionnaire.

Regarding feelings of powerlessness for the two groups, Kafka's (1986) findings indicated "there was a significant difference in feelings of hopefulness regarding the delivery experience based on the type of birth. Fathers whose wives had a vaginal delivery felt significantly more hopeful than fathers whose wives had a cesarean delivery at the $p<.05$ level of significance" (p. 48). No significant differences were found between the means of the two delivery groups with regard to the fathers' feelings of control and contentment with decisions made concerning the pregnancy and delivery period.

Other results denoted that 96 percent of all fathers responding strongly agreed or agreed that decisions were made with their wives during pregnancy and delivery. Ninety-four percent of the fathers had questions before or during the delivery, with fathers of cesarean births indicating 13 percent more satisfaction with how the questions were answered. Ninety-four percent of all fathers in the study understood information given to them with 100 percent of the fathers of cesarean births expressing that the information helped them with the birthing experience compared to 91 percent of the vaginal delivery fathers indicating the information had been helpful.

Fathers who were able to make decisions with their wives and others and understood the information given to them felt more control (power) than those fathers who did not. There were no significant differences in relationship to the timing of when questions were asked or answered on powerlessness. One of the major conclusions of this study was that the more information that was understood, the more powerful the fathers felt.

Kafka's (1986) results contribute to the developing knowledge base concerning new fathers' birth experiences, conceptualized as a developmental life change. "The cognitive, emotional, and social human responses of the two groups of fathers assisted in giving some basis for further understanding of fathers' feelings concerning their childbirth experiences," (pp. ii–iii).

Gale-Swanson (1986) conducted a study focusing on a different developmental life change and associated human responses. This study documented health behaviors and factors that influence health behaviors in elderly individuals. In this descriptive study, Gale-Swanson used the framework developed by Loomis and Wood (1983) for two reasons. "First, the model's third dimension of clinical decision making allows for the assessment of human responses to actual or potential health problems. Second, the model identified six human response systems that closely resemble health behaviors (Gochman,

1982)," (p. 7). For this study, the potential health problem was identified as the developmental life change of aging. Hence, the assessment component of data collection focused on identifying human responses associated with the developmental life change of aging through the identification of health behaviors and the factors that influence health behaviors (see Figure 4).

In order to successfully integrate the Loomis/Wood Model and the concept of health behavior in this study, the term *potential health problem* was altered to *potential health challenge* because of the need to continue the incorporation of the positive aspect of health in the nursing framework. The incorporation of health allowed for the presence of strengthening and limiting components which result from interaction of various factors (American Nurses' Association, 1980). "The developmental life change of aging was therefore recognized as a potential health challenge because of the inherent ability for this life process to exhibit strengthening and/or limiting attributes" (Gale-Swanson, 1986, p. 9).

For this study, the convenience sample was comprised of 20 female and male participants, who were 65 years and older and not participating in a regular work situation. Participants resided either in a semi-independent/retirement living accommodation, or an independent living arrangement. Participants were oriented to time, place, and person; demonstrated adequate hearing, vision, and hand coordination; and needed to be involved in their usual (typical) activities during the study.

Data were collected by use of two questionnaires and the Experience Sampling Method (ESM). Electronic pagers were sounded once during every two-hour period by the investigator, between the hours of 8 AM and 10 PM, every day for one week, signalling participants to complete a Participant Activity Sheet (PAS). A total of 49 PASs and one Post Survey Questionnaire (PSQ) were completed by each participant. The data were described by frequency distributions and percentages.

Gale-Swanson's (1986) results indicated that these elderly: exercised a variety of overt behaviors and thoughts; experienced primarily positive emotions; often had expectations of an activity which, for the most part, were fulfilled; valued their activities; and engaged in the activity by themselves at home. Such study findings attested to the existence of many types of health behavior human responses and factors that influenced health behaviors in the elderly, all fitting within the framework of Loomis and Wood.

Figure 4
Gale-Swanson's Integrated Model for the Study of
Health Behaviors of Elderly Individuals

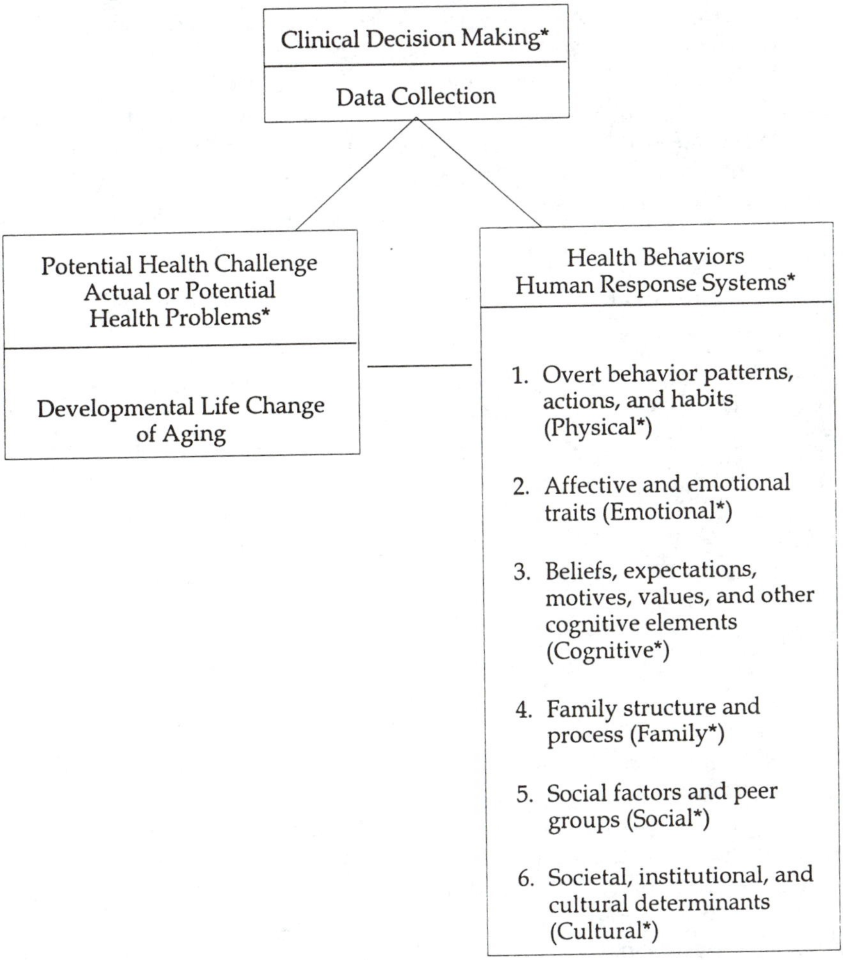

Clinical Decision Making*
Data Collection

Potential Health Challenge Actual or Potential Health Problems*	Health Behaviors Human Response Systems*
Developmental Life Change of Aging	1. Overt behavior patterns, actions, and habits (Physical*)
	2. Affective and emotional traits (Emotional*)
	3. Beliefs, expectations, motives, values, and other cognitive elements (Cognitive*)
	4. Family structure and process (Family*)
	5. Social factors and peer groups (Social*)
	6. Societal, institutional, and cultural determinants (Cultural*)

• Loomis and Wood's Dimensions.

The preceding examples illustrate the utility of the Loomis/Wood Model in providing a content framework for nursing studies. Other researchers have also investigated phenomena resulting from selection of concepts from the interrelated axes of the model. Among these are Woodruff's (1985) study of the prevalence of bulemic human responses in female undergraduate students, and Vanderwalker's (1984) investigation of the communication ability human responses to the acute health deviation of cerebrovascular accident and their association to quality of nursing care. All such studies build upon and contribute knowledge regarding the current definition of nursing proposed and accepted by the American Nurses Association (1980).

Research Using Loomis and Wood's Four Prototypes

In their initial article describing the model, Loomis and Wood (1983) posited the existence of "four prototypes of health care situations" (p. 5). These health care situations define the contexts within which nursing is practiced and allow for important temporal distinctions among the content elements of the model. They offer additional avenues for investigating nursing phenomena through examination of interrelationships of concepts within the two content axes of the model. Moreover, the prototypes give helpful guidance for investigations regarding planning, treatment, and evaluation as part of clinical decision making. The four prototypes include those in which: (1) health problems precede human responses; (2) human responses precede health problems; (3) health problems are defined by human responses; and (4) health problems interact with human responses (see Figure 5).

The first prototype, in which health problems precede human responses, most often signifies a situation in which an acute health deviation occurs yielding certain human responses which follow. This prototype usually is aligned with the medical model where the major focus is on the acute health deviation such as influenza or physical injury and on efforts to deter or eliminate invasive organisms or repair damage caused by trauma. Collaborative nurse-physician interventions are targeted to the correcting of physiological damage and the minimizing of further physical complications. The primary and initial concern is usually on the actual health problem and the physical human response system. The secondary concerns most often

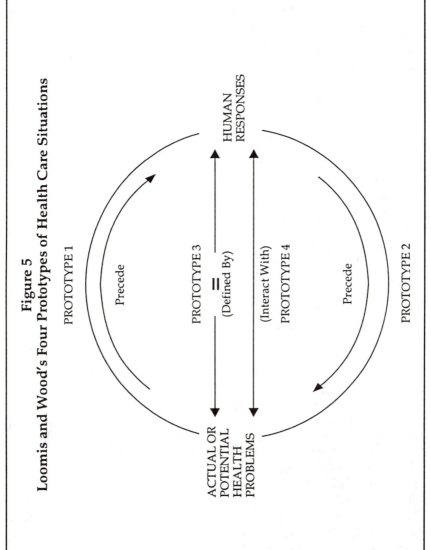

Figure 5
Loomis and Wood's Four Prototypes of Health Care Situations

are the emotional, cognitive, and family human response systems and other human responses.

In the second prototype Loomis and Wood (1983) identify, human responses precede actual or potential health problems. The nursing focus is on the human responses which may presuppose actual or potential health problems. Beliefs or mores regarding aging or illness which may influence an individual's response to an actual or potential health problem such as the developmental life change of retirement or an acute health deviation such as flu exemplify such cultural factors.

The third prototype Loomis and Wood (1983) identify is actual and potential health problems as defined by human responses. Here the nursing focus is independent nursing action to alleviate or ameliorate the human responses defining the actual and potential health problems. Fever of unknown origin or the diagnostic categories of the *Diagnostic and Statistical Manual of Mental Disorders* of the American Psychiatric Association (1980) exemplify actual or potential health problems as defined by human responses.

Loomis and Wood (1983) identify the fourth prototype as actual and potential health problems which interact with human responses. Here the focus of treatment is equal attention to the human responses as well as to the actual or potential health problems. Chronic health problems such as diabetes and chronic obstructive pulmonary disease (COPD) are examples of this prototype. The effectiveness of the treatments for chronic health deviations require the cooperation of patients and their willingness to change.

In general, the four prototypes assist nurses in more clearly defining the health care situations at hand. Further, they can assist nurses in developing their research from among clinical decision-making alternatives that may be collaborative or independent in nature. For instance, when investigations determine that certain actual or potential health problems consistently lead to specific patterns of human responses, prescriptive research can be initiated whereby nurses and physicians collaborate to alleviate temporary physiological imbalances and correct negative physical responses. When human responses precede health problems, nursing research can focus on nursing action to prevent potential health problems from occurring. When research indicates health problems are defined by human responses, nurses can examine independent strategies to decrease the problematic nature of human responses, symptoms, and behaviors. Finally, when health problems are interactive with human responses, nursing clinical decision-making inquiry can emphasize research in which nurses assist patients/clients in self-regulation of their human responses.

Nursing research focusing on the evaluation aspect of the clinical decision-making axis of the Loomis/Wood Model would be the next logical step, once prescriptive research had been proposed or conducted. Evaluation research of this type would converge on "cure" as conceptualized by Loomis and Wood (1983). A positive evaluation outcome of cure could be operationalized for each of the four prototypes as follows:

1. When actual health problems precede human responses, cure is defined as readjustment of the temporary physiologic/physical imbalance and patient and support systems coping with the acute health deviations.
2. When human responses precede health problems, cure is evidenced by smooth developmental and environmental transitions and the absence of abnormal physical, emotional, and other responses.
3. When health problems are defined by human responses, cure would be defined and documented most often in terms of physiologic, emotional, cognitive, social, and other human responses which are nonproblematic.
4. When health problems are interactive with human response systems, cure is measured by the effective management of the chronic health deviation with minimal disruption to the person's personal, professional, family, and social functioning, and in repatterning of human responses.

Nurse researchers have focused a considerable amount of energy into selecting conceptual frameworks for organization of nursing research studies. This section has shown that the Loomis/Wood Model is a compelling and attractive framework, useful for organizing nursing knowledge and abstractly guiding research in clinical nursing. Using the Loomis/Wood Model, many research purposes can be fulfilled.

In addition, through the generation and classification of nursing diagnoses, description or factor isolating can be accomplished (Dickoff, James, & Wiedenbach, 1968). Studies examining relationships between particular actual or potential health problems and specific human responses are factor relating. Relationships between

72 JOAN STEHLE WERNER

Figure 6
Integration of Lazarus and Folkman's Stress Theory with the Loomis/Wood Model

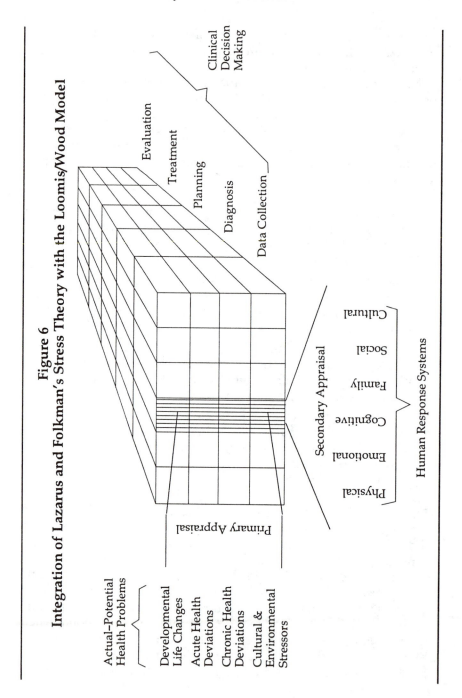

Figure 7
Rock's Integrated Model for the Study of Cultural Human Responses of Male Hmong

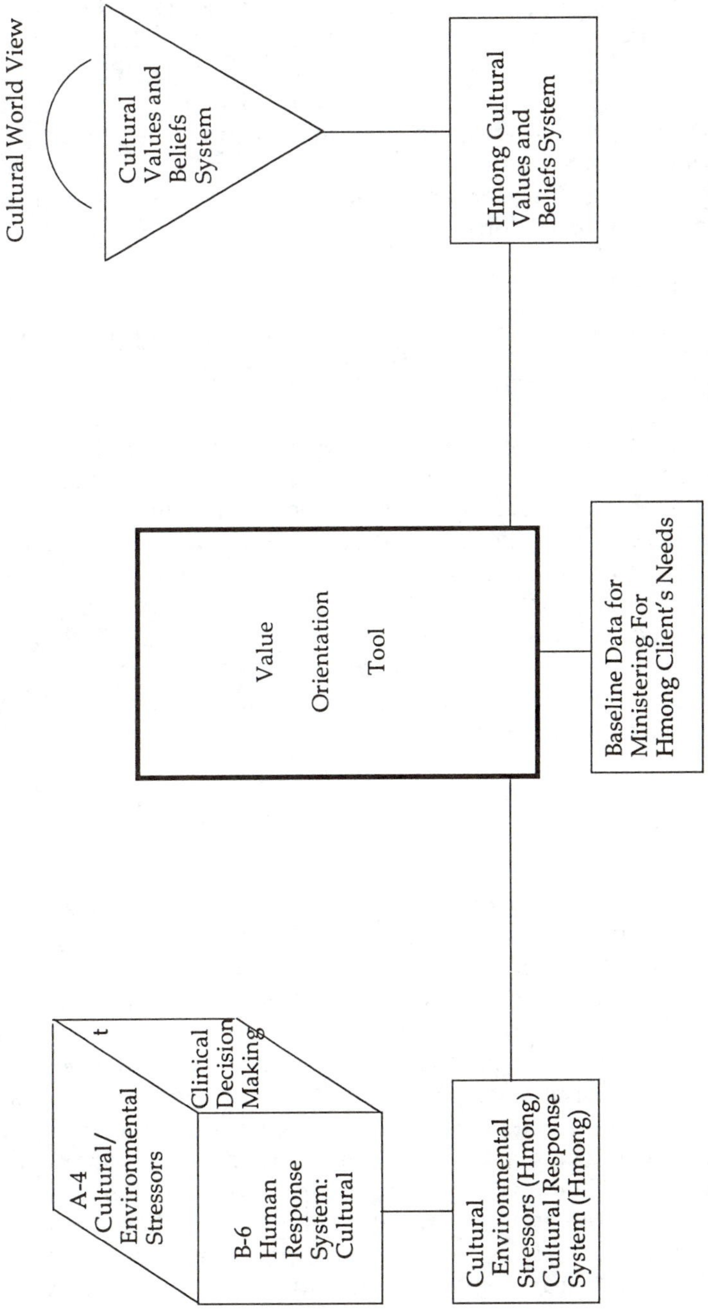

actual and potential health problem categories and human response patterns can be conceptualized as situation relating. Situation-producing research can also be conducted using this model. This research is prescriptive because it indicates the outcomes to be produced (cure) and abstract because it indicates the means for producing such situations (treatment). The areas to be given attention in producing cure include relationships or interactions of actual or potential health problems and human responses.

RESEARCH ARTICULATING THE LOOMIS/WOOD MODEL WITH EXISTING THEORIES

The case examples in the preceding section demonstrate that most research already conducted using the Loomis/Wood Model has been descriptive, correlational, or exploratory in nature. While these types of research probably flow best from an abstract conceptual framework such as the model at hand, this model is also able to support theory-based research. Theories, whether they be unique to nursing, shared, or borrowed (Johnson, 1968; Stevens, 1984), can be introduced and embedded into various cubicles or sections of the model, and used to address various aspects of a research problem from a deductive perspective.

Borrowed Theory

Borrowed theory, defined as use by nursing of a theory from another discipline without being adapted to nursing and to nursing's concept of man (Johnson, 1968; Stevens, 1984), can be very useful in guiding studies involving any of the actual or potential health problem categories or patterns of human responses from the human response systems axis. For instance, if a researcher was interested in studying human responses associated with a specific acute illness episode, Lazarus and Folkman's (1984) cognitive stress theory could be borrowed and employed. The stress appraisals associated with any of the actual or potential health problem categories could be conceptualized as a threat, harm/loss, or challenge, and these appraisals would be assessed. The associated human responses, arising most likely in the cognitive and emotional human response systems, would also be investigated to establish whether or not stress was associated with this acute illness. Secondary appraisal measures involving several of the human response systems could also be addressed (see Figure 6). Resulting information would be useful both in the domains of psychology and nursing. In this way, various theories and research results based on borrowed theoretical research can be useful in developing a knowledge base within a conceptual framework that encompasses the domain of nursing knowledge. The long-term goal would be to develop nursing clinical decision-making processes that would assist these individuals with stress.

Shared Theory

Just as borrowed theory can be integrated into the model for research purposes, so too shared theory or less abstract conceptual models can be employed in order to conduct deductive research. Shared theory is theory adapted from other disciplines which has been modified and applied in the nursing milieu (Stevens, 1984). Several of the newer, middle-range theories and frameworks, many of which have been developed through qualitative research strategies, can be infused within the model in order to yield information useful not only to nurses but also to other disciplines (see, for example, works by Carter, 1989; Phillips & Rampusheski, 1986; and Van Dongen, 1990).

Case example.   Rock (1987) has conducted a shared theory study designed to identify the cultural human responses of male members of the Hmong community in a mid-sized Wisconsin city in terms of their cultural values and beliefs. The long-term goal of this program of research was to enable nurses to intervene effectively in supporting Hmong individuals and families, as well as community networks.

For this study, conceptual frameworks involved the more abstract Loomis/Wood Model in combination with Leininger's (1984) Sunrise Model. The focus of the actual or potential health problem at hand was Cultural/Environmental Stressors of the Hmong. According to Rock (1987), the "Hmong community may be experiencing struggle in assimilating into American society" (p. 11). In terms of the Human Response System category, Rock examined the Cultural Human Response which was further conceptualized using Leininger's Sunrise Model (see Figure 7).

Utilizing a value orientation assessment tool, the participants were asked to select items on a 22-item ordinal scale questionnaire based on the rural scale by Kluckhohn (Kluckhohn & Murray, 1950). The 20 male participants responded to hypothetical questions involving four of the following value orientations: activity, relational roles, time, and man-nature. The male Hmong's responses maintained that in three value orientations—activity, relational roles, and man-nature—the responses contrasted with dominant Anglo-Saxon American value orientation preferences. This study provided a beginning understanding of baseline values of the Hmong culture of those living in the Midwest, and provided knowledge about the Hmong cultural human responses to cultural environmental stressors.

Unique Theory

Unique nursing theory is theory developed within and for the disciplinary matrix (Fawcett, 1984; Johnson, 1968) of nursing. The Loomis/Wood Model articulates well with most of the dominant nursing theories, and these theories can be used to guide research flowing from the model. Most nursing theories, particularly those by "Needs Theorists" (Meleis, 1985, p. 172) such as Abdellah, Henderson, and Orem, can be integrated with aspects of the model to study both nursing clinical decision making and particular phenomena.

For example, with Orem's (1980) theory, classified as a needs theory by Meleis, Universal, Developmental and Health Deviation Requisites/Needs can be conceptualized as fitting within the Actual or Potential Health Problem axis. Self-care Capabilities and Demands can be thought of as fitting within Human Response Systems, as can Self-Care Agency. To eliminate the deficit between self-care capabilities and demand, clinical decision making along the process axis is employed, and the process can be further categorized as wholly compensatory, partly compensatory, or supportive-educative (Orem, 1980, p. 96) (see Figure 8). Using the Loomis/Wood Model, then, in combination with a unique nursing theory can contribute knowledge not only regarding content but through studying particular clinical decision-making processes as well.

Interaction theories (Meleis, 1985, p. 174) are also well suited for adaptation and use with the Loomis/Wood Model. Most of these theories fit best within the process axis of the model and they specify

Figure 8
Integration of Orem's Theory with Loomis/Wood Model

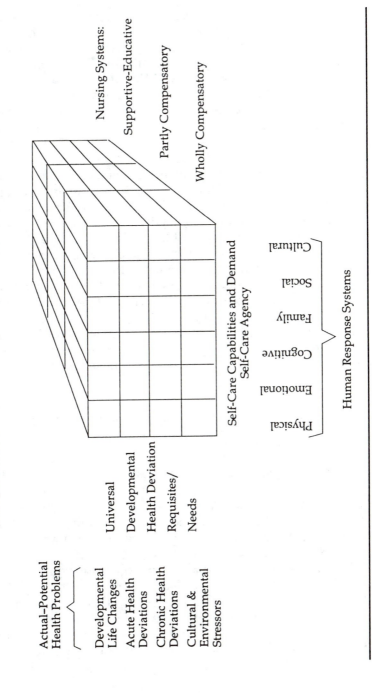

how the process of clinical decision making can be carried out. For example, with King's (1981) theory, the goals established by nurse and patient may refer to actual or potential health problems and human responses as specified on both content axes of the Loomis/ Wood Model. The process axis of the model, however, would be replaced with the processes of action, reaction, and interaction whereby nurse and patient interact for goal attainment (see Figure 9).

Indeed, those theories Meleis (1985) refers to as "Outcome Theories" (p. 179) also articulate well with the cubicular framework. Theories and concepts developed by these theorists most often provide the specifics of the content axes, and occasionally contribute to the outcome aspect of the process axis. For instance, with Levine's (1971) theory, the four principles of energy, personal integrity, structural integrity, and social integrity can replace subconcepts of the Actual or Potential Health Problem axis, while the organismic responses of fear, inflammation, stress, and sensory responses directly reflect certain patterns of human responses both within and among Human Response System categories. Levine's concepts of Conservation of Energy and Integrity, as well as restoration of activity and well-being, form goals or outcomes for the process axis (see Figure 10).

The preceding examples depict the flexibility of the Loomis/Wood Model for use with various theories. Further creative integrations of particular theories with this model seem nearly limitless.

RESEARCH WITH THE LOOMIS/WOOD MODEL
FROM PARADIGMATIC PERSPECTIVES

In clinical nursing research, the uses of the Loomis/Wood Model already described in most cases have been implemented using a deductive mode of inquiry. The studies previously cited illustrate the flexibility of application of the model emerging from positivism (Reese, 1980) or the positive-empiricist paradigmatic tradition (Woods & Catanzaro, 1988).

The investigations described in the former section of this chapter could further be characterized as: (1) "factor isolating" (Dickoff, James, & Wiedenbach, 1968, p. 419)—identifying characteristics of a particular actual or potential health problem or specific human responses; (2) "factor relating" (Dickoff et al., p. 419)—establishing particular groupings of related human responses; (3) "situation relat-

Figure 9
Integration of King's Theory with Loomis/Wood Model

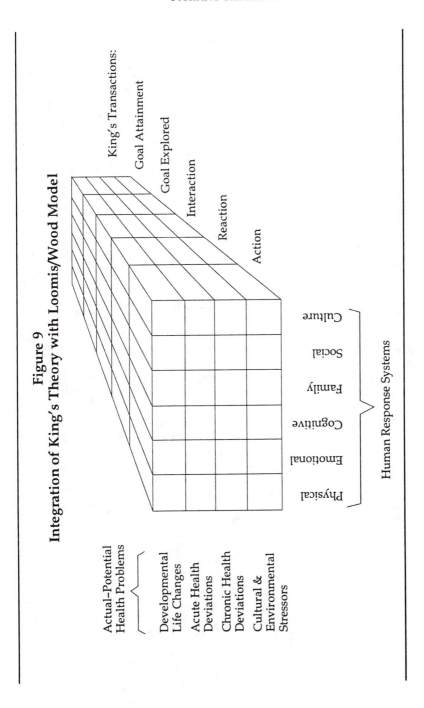

Figure 10
Integration of Levine's Theory with Loomis/Wood Model

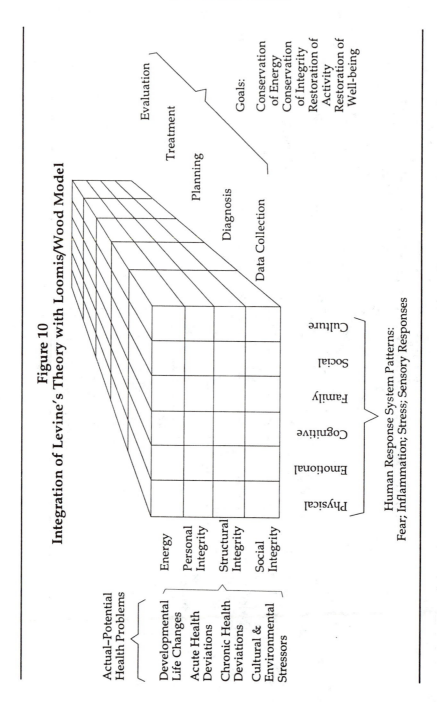

ing" (Dickoff et al., p. 420)—discovering various patterns between one or more actual or potential health problems and constellations of human responses; and (4) "situation-producing" (Dickoff et al., p. 420)—incorporation of the clinical decision-making process axis to carry out certain nursing prescriptions and to examine their outcomes. All of these types of research are presumed to be deductive in nature flowing from a paradigmatic perspective which espouses prediction and control as well as understanding and explanation.

On the other hand, according to Woods and Catanzaro (1988), "The naturalistic-inductive paradigm is derived from a tradition that assumes that facts and principles are embedded in both historical and cultural contexts. Truth is seen as dynamic and derived from human interaction with real social and historical settings" (p. 23). The inductive types of research, most often utilizing the various qualitative methods, are generally conducted in natural environments and often employ several data collection strategies.

Major kinds of naturalistic-inductive research include grounded theory (Chenitz & Swanson, 1986; Glaser & Strauss, 1967; Stern, 1980), ethnography (Leininger, 1985), and phenomenological investigation (Davies, 1973; Swanson-Kauffman & Schonwald, 1988). Usually, with any of these research designs, the ultimate goal is understanding or explanation. In addition, all generally begin with a phenomenon of interest, or at least a notion regarding an arena of concern for examination. The Loomis/Wood Model can give direction to the selection of phenomena of interest in that Actual or Potential Health Problems and Human Responses provide extensive boundaries, within which most events or experiences which accommodate with nursing's realm of knowledge comply. Within these boundaries, a "focus for the inquiry" (Lincoln & Guba, 1985, p. 226) or a problem can be identified. In addition, for these studies, the third axis of the model could be replaced with a third content dimension. This axis (see Figure 11) could be designed to capture settings which are believed to be integral to knowledge within this paradigm. Categories within this axis might include historical, social, and possibly other setting influences believed to be integral to knowledge.

The Naturalistic Inductive Paradigm

Case example. Smith (1988) conducted a study which, in part, identified actual or potential health problems and human responses of Chinese women living in the United States (see Figure 12). The pertinent research questions focused on understanding of the experiences of these women, and were broad questions bounded only by the concepts of human responses and actual or potential health problems.

Data were collected by means of long interviews from a convenience sample of ten Chinese women living in a large metropolitan city on the West Coast of the United States. An entrée (Lonner & Berry, 1986) accompanied the researcher to all women's homes and also served as a translator for those women who did not speak English well, or at all. Qualitative responses were content analyzed.

The majority of responses, which are too comprehensive for inclusion here, were an integration of cultural human responses and actual and potential health problems. The women described and discussed their perceptions using a mixture of Western and Chinese concepts, theories, and terminology. The basis for choice of Chinese or Western health care depended on the severity of the health problem.

Through analysis of responses it was found that "generation" was an important theme for these women, perhaps an important delineation of the Settings axis of the modified model as portrayed in Figure 11. The similarities and differences in the identified cultural human responses were then compared based on generation. Similarities between the older and younger generations were found in their perceptions of health, actual health deviations, whom they sought for advice for health concerns, use of Eastern physicians, expectation for care of aging parents, and preferred method of support. Differences between the generations were found in their body language, speech pattern, eating habits, effects of health deviation on their families, awareness of a health deviation, support system, chronic health deviations, perception of health promotion, and care of aging parents.

This immediate example illustrates again the utility of the Loomis/Wood Model, even with studies stemming from a naturalistic perspective. A major reason for such flexibility is this: the model is constructed from sweeping constructs, which in concert establish boundaries for content based on the currently most widely accepted definition of nursing. Hopefully, the tremendous advantages of this model for application in research has become vivid for the reader. Other researchers' creative use of the model will doubtless lead to many more inventively designed applications in nursing inquiry.

Figure 11
Loomis/Wood Model Modified for Use with Qualitative Research

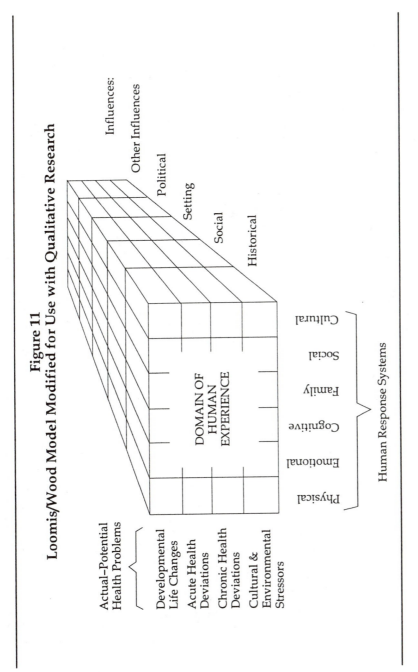

Figure 12

Model for the Study of Cultural Human Responses of Chinese Women Adapted from the Model for the Study of Clinical Nursing

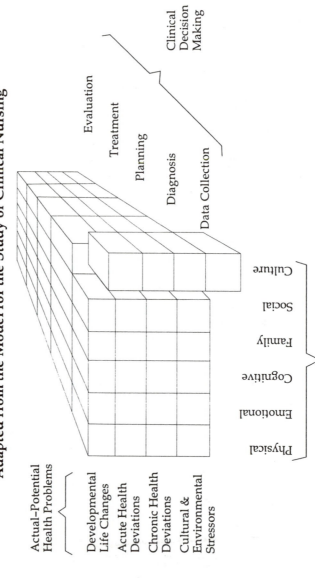

From "Cure: The Potential Outcome of Nursing Care," by M. Loomis and D. Wood, *Image 15*, p. 4. Reprinted by permission.

CONCLUSION

Nurse researchers have focused a considerable amount of energy and effort in the selection of conceptual or theoretical frameworks with which to organize clinical nursing research studies. The Loomis/Wood Model, first described in their 1983 article, "Cure: The Potential Outcomes of Nursing Care," provides an attractive alternative for individuals who are involved in the process of identifying a framework for organizing how they view the profession of nursing and its unique body of knowledge.

Particularly attractive features of this model as an organizing framework for nursing research include: (1) the ease of articulation of the Loomis/Wood Model with the American Nurses' Association (1980) definition of nursing; (2) the articulation of the Loomis/Wood Model with the taxonomy of nursing diagnoses established by the North American Nursing Diagnosis Association; and (3) the easy articulation the Loomis/Wood Model has with several nursing theoretical frameworks. In this chapter, several uses of the model have been delineated. Among these uses are research designs flowing from the positivist-empiricist paradigm including, but not limited to, descriptive, exploratory, correlational, comparative, quasi-experimental, and experimental research. It has also been proposed that the model may have utility for conducting qualitative research.

Since 1983, University of Wisconsin-Eau Claire students (undergraduate and graduate) and colleagues in research, practice, and education have applied and validated the usefulness of the model as an organizing framework for at least 12 research studies having a clinical nursing focus. In most cases, the model has been tested utilizing a deductive mode of inquiry, although the use of inductive methodologies is equally possible. To date, we have yet to experience a negative case in which the model has not been applicable. The studies already completed show the model's utility in clinical research. Perhaps other researchers will yet devise even more insightful functions for this obviously salient framework.

REFERENCES

American Nurses' Association. (1980). *Nursing: A social policy statement.* New York: Author.

American Psychiatric Association. (1980). *Diagnostic and statistical manual of mental disorders, (3rd ed.)*. Washington, DC: Author.

Anderson, J. (1982). The significance of hunger to nursing. In C. M. Norris (Ed.), *Concept clarification in nursing*. Rockville, MD: Aspen Systems, 199–222.

Carter, S. L. (1989). Themes of grief. *Nursing Research, 38*, 354–358.

Chenitz, W. C., & Swanson, J. M. (1986). *From practice to grounded theory*. Menlo Park, CA: Addison-Wesley.

Davis, A. J. (1973). The phenomenological approach in nursing research. In E. A. Garrison (Ed.), *Doctoral preparation for nurses with emphasis on the psychiatric field*. San Francisco: University of California, 212–228.

Dickoff, J., James, P., & Wiedenbach, E. (1968). Theory in a practice discipline: Part I. Practice oriented theory. *Nursing Research, 17*, 420–425.

Dubin, R. (1978). *Theory building, revised edition*. New York: The Free Press.

Fawcett, J. (1984). The metaparadigm of nursing: present status and future refinements. *Image: The Journal of Nursing Scholarship, 16*(3), 84–87.

Flaskerud, J. H., & Halloran, E. (1980). Areas of agreement in nursing theory development. *Advances in Nursing Science, 3*(1), 1–7.

Gale-Swanson, E. (1986). *Health behaviors and the factors that influence health behaviors in an elderly population*. Unpublished master's thesis, University of Wisconsin-Eau Claire.

Glaser, B. & Strauss, A. (1967). *The discovery of grounded theory*. Chicago: Adline.

Gochman, D. S. (1982). Labels, systems and motives: Some perspectives for future research and programs. *Health Education Quarterly, 9*(2 & 3), 167/263–174/270.

Gortner, S. R. (1990). Nursing values and science: Toward a science philosophy. *Image: Journal of Nursing Scholarship, 22*, 101–105.

Henderson, V. (1964). The nature of nursing. *American Journal of Nursing, 64*(8), 62–68.

Henderson, V. (1966). *The nature of nursing*. New York: Macmillan.

Johnson, D. E. (1968). Theory in nursing: Borrowed and unique. *Nursing Research, 17*, 206–207.

Johnson, S. E. (1989). Sleep pattern disturbance: Defining characteristics observable in practice. In R. M. Carroll-Johnson (Ed.), *Classification of nursing diagnoses: Proceedings of the Eighth Conference*. Philadelphia: Lippincott, 368–370.

Kafka, E. A. (1986). *The concept of powerlessness among fathers involved with the birth experience*. Unpublished master's thesis, University of Wisconsin-Eau Claire.

King, I. (1981). *A theory for nursing: Systems, concepts, process*. New York: John Wiley & Sons.

Kluckhohn, C., & Murray, H. (1950). *Personality in nature, society, and culture*. New York: Knopf.

Kuznar, K. A. (1988). *The important needs of family members of critically ill patients.* Unpublished master's thesis, University of Wisconsin-Eau Claire.

Leininger, M. (1984). *Care, the essence of nursing and health.* Thorofare, NJ: Slack.

Leininger, M. M. (Ed.) (1985). *Qualitative research methods in nursing.* Orlando: Grune & Stratton.

Levine, M. E. (1971). Holistic nursing. *Nursing Clinics of North America, 6*(2), 258–263.

Lincoln, Y. S., & Guba, E. (1985). *Naturalistic inquiry.* Beverly Hills: Sage.

Lonner, W., & Berry, J. (1986). *Field methods in cross cultural research.* Beverly Hills: Sage.

Loomis, M., & Wood, D. J. (1983). Cure: the potential outcome of nursing care. *Image: The Journal of Nursing Scholarship, 15*(1), 4–7.

MacLean, S. L. (1989). Activity intolerance: Cues for diagnosis. In R. N. Carroll-Johnson (Ed.), *Classification of nursing diagnoses: Proceedings of the Eighth Conference.* Philadelphia: Lippincott, 320–327.

Mahoney, K. (1989). A validation study of the nursing diagnosis potential for infection. In R. M. Carroll-Johnson (Ed.), *Classification of nursing diagnoses: Proceedings of the Eighth Conference.* Philadelphia: Lippincott, 333–340.

Meleis, A. I. (1985). *Theoretical nursing: Development and progress.* Philadelphia: Lippincott.

Norris, C. M. (1982). *Concept clarification in nursing.* Rockville, MD: Aspen Systems.

Oleson, M. A. (1984). *A study of observable manifestations and subjective responses of fatigue in adult female patients having elective abdominal surgery.* Unpublished master's thesis, University of Wisconsin-Eau Claire.

Orem, D. E. (1980). *Nursing: Concepts of practice,* 2nd edition. New York: McGraw-Hill.

Paremski, A. F. (1989). *A comparison of traditional methods of pain alleviation with patient controlled analgesia in orthopedic surgical patients.* Unpublished master's thesis, University of Wisconsin-Eau Claire.

Phillips, L. R., & Rempusheski. (1986). Caring for the frail elderly at home: Toward a theoretical explanation of the dynamics of poor quality family caregiving. *Advances in Nursing Science, 8*(4), 62–84.

Reese, W. L. (1980). *Dictionary of philosophy and religion.* Atlantic Highlands, NJ: Humanities.

Rock, J. M. (1987). *A value orientation used as a cultural assessment tool for family members of the Hmong community.* Unpublished master's theses, University of Wisconsin-Eau Claire.

Schams, K. A. (1988). *Social support of bulemic women in treatment.* Unpublished master's thesis, University of Wisconsin-Eau Claire.

Schultz, P. R., & Meleis, A. (1988). Nursing epistology: Traditions, insights, questions. *Image: Journal of Nursing Scholarship, 20,* 217–221.

Silko, B. J. (1985). *A study of employed adult women's concerns regarding health, education, family, self, and career.* Unpublished master's thesis, University of Wisconsin-Eau Claire.

Smith, A. (1988). *Identifiable cultural human responses of Chinese women to actual and potential health problems.* Unpublished master's thesis, University of Wisconsin-Eau Claire.

Smith, S. K. (1988). An analysis of the phenomenon of deterioration in the critically ill. *Image: The Journal of Nursing Scholarship, 21*(1), 12–15.

Sperstad, R. A. (1988). *Physical comfort and self-esteem of pregnant women who participated in a structured maternity fitness program and pregnant women who attended prenatal education class.* Unpublished master's thesis, University of Wisconsin-Eau Claire.

Stern, P. N. (1980). Grounded theory methodology: Its uses and processes. *Image, 12*(1), 20–23.

Stevens, B. J. (1984). *Nursing theory: Analysis, application, evaluation,* second edition. Boston: Little, Brown.

Swanson, E., & McCloskey, J. (1986). Publishing opportunities for nurses. *Nursing Outlook, 34,* 227.

Swanson-Kauffman, K., & Schonwald, E. (1988). Phenomenology. In B. Sarter (Ed.), *Paths to knowledge: Innovative research methods for nursing.* New York: National League for Nursing, 97–105.

University of Wisconsin-Eau Claire Nursing Faculty. (1984). *Faculty Handbook.* Eau Claire, WI: Author.

Van Dongen, C. J. (1990). Agonizing questioning: Experience of survivors of suicide victims. *Nursing Research, 39,* 224–255.

Vanderwalker, J. (1984). *Communication ability: Its association with the quality of nursing care received by aphasic cerebrovascular accident patients.* Unpublished master's thesis. University of Wisconsin-Eau Claire.

Watson, J. (1988). *Nursing: Human science and human care—a theory of nursing.* New York: National League for Nursing.

Webster, G., Jacox, A., & Baldwin, B. (1981). Nursing theory and the ghost of the received view. In J. C. McCloskey & H. Grace (Eds.). *Current Issues in Nursing.* Oxford: Blackwell Scientific Publications.

Weekes, D. P., & Rankin, S. (1988). Life-span developmental methods: Application to nursing research. *Nursing Research, 37,* 380–383.

Whitley, G. G. (1989). An analysis of the nursing diagnosis anxiety. In R. M. Carroll-Johnson (Ed.). *Classification of nursing diagnoses: Proceedings of the Eighth Conference.* Philadelphia: Lippincott, 371–375.

Woodruff, J. M. (1985). *A descriptive study of the prevalence of self-reported bulemic behaviors in female undergraduate students.* Unpublished master's thesis. University of Wisconsin-Eau Claire.

Woods, N. F., & Catanzaro, M. (1988). *Nursing research: Theory and practice.* St. Louis: C. V. Mosby.

4

Application of the Loomis/Wood Model as a Conceptual Framework in Nursing Practice

Joan Stehle Werner

*T*he true test of any conceptual framework for nursing is its utility in nursing practice. Because the Loomis/Wood Model is based on the most widely accepted definition of nursing as forwarded in Nursing Social Policy Statement (ANA, 1980), its relevance to nursing practice is conceived of as having a strong, direct, and applicable link. But, beyond being derived from a definition of nursing, the issue of how nurses can go about using the model in practice needs further clarification. In this chapter, I will describe the utility of the Loomis/Wood Model for nurses and provide both actual and hypothetical examples of its effective use in nursing practice.

Nursing conceptual frameworks can serve many purposes in the practice arena. First, they can guide the nurse clinician through the clinical decision-making process, focusing on a thorough assessment, and pointing to areas for intervention or treatment. A model well suited for this purpose would indicate salient content areas and guide the clinician to examine client data that otherwise might be overlooked or disregarded. A nursing content-specific model could also suggest nursing diagnoses which have been found through research to be present given certain phenomena and circumstances.

Second, nursing conceptual frameworks in practice can organize the roles and functions of groups of nurses. In this way, a particular model can pinpoint the domain and boundaries of practice for either a nursing service dedicated to one major function, or can form the skeletal structure of an organization of nurses performing various diverse functions. In fact, the very term *nursing service organization* suggests the vital inclusion of a nursing-dedicated model used to organize the service, rather than another type of model—for example, the medical model. In addition, a model can serve to illumine foci of independent nursing practice, interdependent nursing practice, and dependent nursing practice.

Third, a particular nursing conceptual model in practice can be of significant aid in the engineering of the principal components of a specialty nursing practice. As society changes, as technologies develop further, as knowledge expands, and as public needs for nursing increase, nursing conceptual models can steer the course of providing a holistic approach to health care for a segment of society. A model that specifies areas of unique concern to nursing can serve to highlight certain domains which can be targeted as spheres of specialty practice. This specialty practice may be implemented by nurse entrepreneurs, clinical nurse specialists, or by nurse practitioners.

As indicated above, the major purposes for a conceptual framework in nursing practice provide only three of several potential functions of models in nursing practice. It is probably true that nursing has yet to develop fully all of the uses of conceptual models as it serves society. The three major functions proposed, however, will serve as the structure of this chapter, which supports the use of the Loomis/Wood Model (Loomis & Wood, 1983) specifically in three types of situations: (1) as a guide for individual nursing clinical decision making with clients/patients; (2) as a framework for organization of nursing service; and (3) as a guide to domains for specialty nursing practice. Illustrations for each of these proposed functions with examples of actual or hypothetical applicaton of the Loomis and Wood framework for practice will be included.

THE LOOMIS/WOOD MODEL IN NURSING CLINICAL DECISION MAKING

The Loomis/Wood Model provides an exemplary utilitarian framework in nursing practice by virtue of the fact that it arose from the currently most well-accepted definition of nursing. Developed by the American Nurses' Association (ANA) (1980), this definition professes that nursing "is the diagnosis and treatment of human responses to actual or potential health problems" (p. 10) (see Figure 1). This ANA document further states that this definition of nursing "points to four defining characteristics of nursing: phenomena, theory application, nursing action, and evaluation of effects of action in relation to phenomena" (p. 10). All such characteristics are clearly central to the Loomis/Wood Model where phenomena are represented by the intersection of actual and potential health problems with human responses; where theory application is implied as the means by which the phenomena are understood and interpreted and by which the nurse determines appropriate actions; and where nursing action and evaluation of these actions are represented by the clinical decision-making axis (see Figure 2).

But how does the practice of nursing become initiated? Here too the Loomis/Wood Model is illustrative. According to the ANA (1980), nursing is directed to the "(1) reactions of individuals and groups to actual health problems (health restoring responses), such as the impact of illness effects upon the self and family, and related self-care needs; and (2) concerns of individuals and groups about potential health problems (health supporting responses . . ." (pp. 10–11). The vertical or first axis of the Loomis/Wood Model portrays four dimensions of actual or potential health problems which often, when experienced or perceived by persons, places them in a context of requiring nursing care. The four categories included in this dimension are: (1) Developmental Life Changes, (2) Acute Health Deviations, (3) Chronic Health Deviations, and (4) Cultural and Environmental Stressors (see Figure 1).

A condition such as acute illness, then, could initiate the need for nursing to carry out clinical decision making. The nurse would probably initially focus on assessing, diagnosing, planning, treating, and evaluating treatment of human responses related to the acute health deviation, or acute illness (see Figure 3). The ANA (1980) further specifies that these human responses include: "Any observable manifestation, need, condition, concern, event, dilemma, difficulty, occurrence, or fact that can be described or scientifically explained" (p. 10). As such, the nurse could proceed to assess human responses related to the actual health problem systematically by proceeding through the human response systems and performing appropriate assessment strategies. Once this process had begun, the nurse could

JOAN STEHLE WERNER

Figure 1
Model for the Study of Clinical Nursing

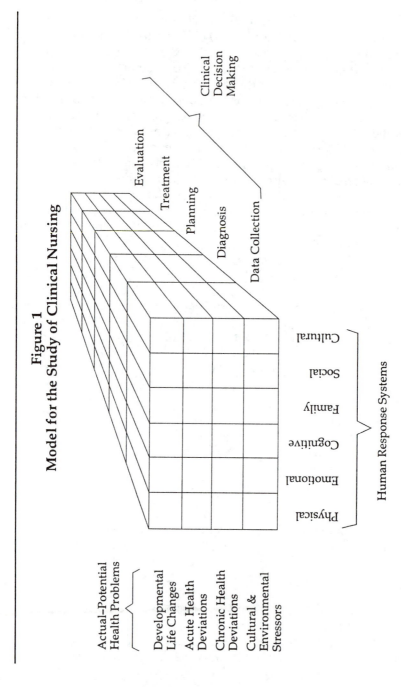

From "Cure: The Potential Outcome of Nursing Care," by M. Loomis and D. Wood, *Image 15*, p. 4. Reprinted by permission.

Figure 2
The Loomis/Wood Model Exemplifying Defining Characteristics of Nursing

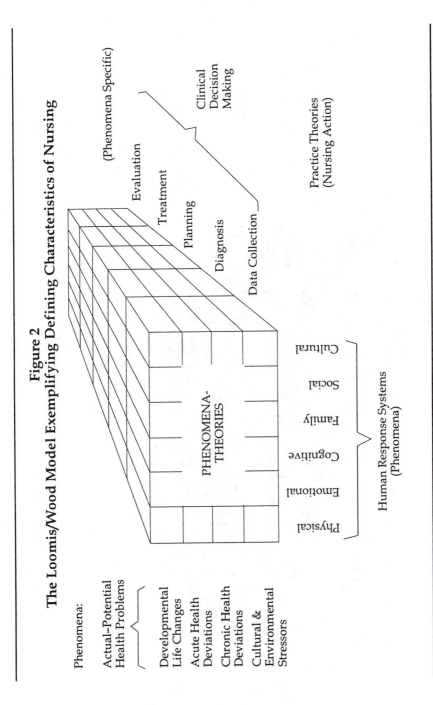

Figure 3
The Loomis/Wood Model as a Guide for Initial Nursing Assessment

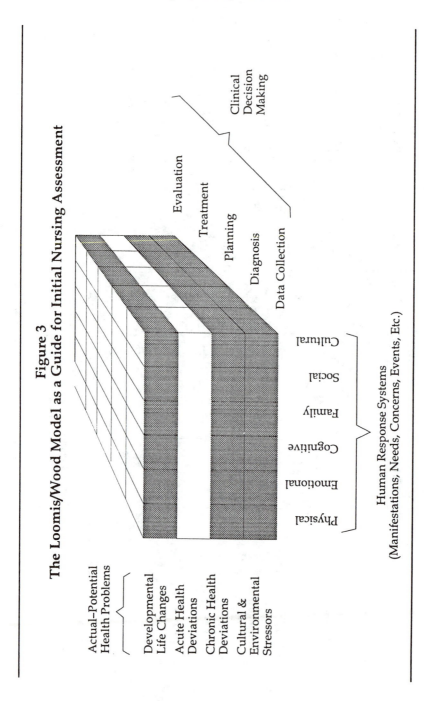

broaden his or her clinical decision making to focus on other actual or potential health problems and the associated human response.

Case Example

An Eau Claire, Wisconsin, hospital developed an intake assessment format for nursing clinical decision making with patients admitted to their facility. This format was based on the Loomis/Wood Model and was designed by a committee of practicing nurses. The information collected was typical of this type of intake assessment, but the organization of the questions and examinations followed the axes, dimensions, and categories of the Loomis/Wood Model. An outline of the assessment/intake process is contained in Table 1.

While this intake assessment process in Table 1 is stated in general terms only, specific questions and observation guides were also developed by the nurses. And, while some of the initial assessment data indicated and collected are similar to those of more traditional nursing admission assessment forms based on the typical review of body systems, it is obvious that the intake information obtained using the Loomis/Wood Model gives a vastly more holistic picture of any individual and his or her problems, needs, and concerns (in other words, his or her human responses) than does a body system assessment. Of course, the nurse also uses his or her knowledge and diagnostic reasoning capabilities (Carnevali, Mitchell, Woods, & Tanner, 1984) to tailor the assessment structure to the individual patient. Yet the format, when used in its entirety, was often found to lead to the discovery of previously unidentified areas of concern to both nurses and patients.

Through use of this assessment process, nurses were able to implement assessment strategies which exemplified all four of the Prototypes of Health Care Situations as specified by Loomis and Wood (1983) (see Figure 4). The first portion of the assessment for these hospitalized patients usually signified the first prototype, "Health problems precede human responses" (p. 5). The focus here was on examining human responses to the actual health problem which led to hospitalization. Often though, through the systematic focus on human responses in all six categories of response systems, nurses identified clusters of human responses which were known to precede certain other health problems—instances of Loomis and Wood's second prototype.

Table 1
Hospital Intake Assessment Outline

I. Identifying Information
II. Actual Health Problems—Reason for admittance to the hospital: (typically an acute health deviation).
  A. Patient's understanding of actual health problem
  B. Patient's understanding of reason for hospitalization
  C. Human responses associated with actual health problem[a,b]
    1. Physical
      a) Questions
      b) Physical assessment if warranted
    2. Emotional
      a) Questions
      b) Observations
    3. Cognitive
      a) Questions
      b) Observations
      c) Mental status examination if warranted
    4. Family
      a) Questions
      b) Observations
      c) Interview of family members if present; if warranted
    5. Social
      a) Questions
      b) Observations
    6. Cultural
      a) Questions
      b) Observations
III. Other Actual or Potential Health Problems
  A. Development Life Changes?
    1. Assessment of Life Change Situations
    2. Assessment of Human Responses via 6 categories
  B. Acute Health Deviations?
    1. Other diseases, physical injury, acute illness, or trauma
    2. Assessment of human responses via 6 categories
  C. Chronic Health Deviations?
    1. Long-standing conditions or diseases
    2. Assessment of Human Responses via 6 categories
  D. Cultural and Environmental Stressors
    1. Health problems
    2. Assessment of Human Responses via 6 categories
IV. Nursing Diagnoses

[a]Specific questions and/or topics for assessment questions were specified.
[b]Behaviors to be observed were specified.

Figure 4
Loomis and Woods' Four Prototypes of Health Care Situations

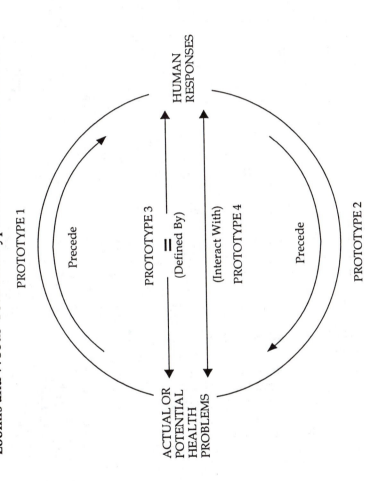

This same focus on human responses throughout the assessment also frequently yielded evidence of health problems defined by human responses, prototype three, or of prototype four, where health problems interact with human responses. Anxiety disorders are illustrative of prototype three, while the interaction of diabetes with lifestyle related practices such as food preference is an example of the prototype four (Loomis & Wood, 1983). The development of the intake assessment based on the Loomis/Wood Model, therefore, has been demonstrated to be an effective method of organizing hospital-based clinical decision-making assessment at least at one facility. Creativity of nurses in other organizations may provide other equally impressive uses for this model in nursing practice.

THE LOOMIS/WOOD MODEL IN THE ORGANIZATION OF NURSING DIAGNOSES

Another significant way in which the Loomis/Wood Model can be extremely serviceable in nursing practice is as an organizing framework for arranging nursing diagnoses into a coherent, understandable, and useful structure. Of course, there are other well-known systems for classifying and organizing nursing diagnoses. However, in the following paragraphs I will propose that the Loomis/Wood Model is a viable alternative to existing schemes that should be considered by those practicing nursing.

The North American Nursing Diagnosis Association (NANDA) has developed one of the most well-known classification systems to portray the logical arrangement of nursing diagnoses. While this organization began by categorizing diagnoses alphabetically, in 1976 NANDA began to employ theory as a base for its taxonomy of diagnostic labels (Gebbie, 1982; Gordon, 1982a,b; Kritek, 1986; Roy, 1984). This approach was used to develop a taxonomy composed of nine human response patterns: Exchanging, Communicating, Relating, Valuing, Choosing, Moving, Perceiving, Knowing, and Feeling (Roy, 1984). These abstract patterns contain a number of applicable diagnoses. According to Kritek (1986), work is continuing on further specifying levels of abstraction associated with each human response pattern.

NANDA's work has been monumental in developing a classification system that will eventually encompass the phenomena of concern to nurses. In reality, however, practicing nurses find the taxonomy confusing and difficult to recall quickly. For example, the categories of communicating and relating are problematic when used by nurses to guide assessment data gathering. Since communication seems a vital part of relating, these two categories do little for a practicing clinician whose goal is to holistically assess the client situation, rather than use his or her cognitive energy to decide how to differentiate the assessment for these two categories. It seems more straightforward and efficacious to group these related diagnoses into a class labeled *social*, as Loomis and Wood do. The label *social* immediately brings to mind both communicating and relating as part of the social realm. Another example of problematic NANDA classifications are the categories of Perceiving, Knowing, and Feeling. Since all knowledge is based on perception, and since feeling and perceiving are often intertwined, these classes of phenomena hold less meaning to a practicing nurse than do Loomis and Wood's Emotional and Cognitive human response systems. Because of the easy recognition of the meaning of Loomis and Wood's categories of human response, they deserve consideration as a method of organizing for nursing diagnoses.

By the same token, Gordon (1982a,b) has also developed an organizing system based on client functioning. Used as a basis for assessment, these Functional Health Patterns include: (1) Health Perception—health management; (2) Nutritional—metabolic, (3) Elimination, (4) Activity—exercise, (5) Sleep—rest, (6) Cognitive—perceptual, (7) Self-perception, (8) Role—relationship, (9) Sexuality—reproductive, (10) Coping—stress tolerance, and (11) Value belief. While this classification system has been found very useful and has been incorporated by others in organizing assessment strategies (for example, see Carpenito, 1987; Maas, Buckwalter, & Hardy, 1991), it too is rather lengthy and complicated. In addition, many of the patterns specified by Gordon focus on bodily function and could be more abstractly grouped for some assessment purposes.

The Loomis/Wood Model is proposed as a classifying scheme that could be developed to circumvent some of the cumbersome qualities of other classification systems. While it is proposed that this system would not replace others developed by NANDA and Gordon, it could serve as an organizer which would be readily understandable to practicing nurses. This proposed system would be built using both the Actual and Potential Health Problem axis and the Human Response System axis of the model. Diagnoses would be situated at the intersection of a Health Problem Classification and a Human Response System. In other words, the sections of the cubicular Loomis/ Wood Model could be superimposed by nursing diagnoses found through research to most likely be operative in the specific situation. An example of the potential outcome of this classification process is illustrated in Figure 5.

In this example, the Actual or Potential Health Problem—Death of Spouse—is categorized under Later Adulthood, which is part of the more abstract category of Developmental Life Changes. Several Human Responses are likely to be engaged surrounding the death of a spouse. Applicable nursing diagnoses might include Dysfunctional grieving; Coping, ineffective, individual; Anxiety; Family processes, altered; and Social isolation, among others. It is evident that these diagnoses tend to indicate the interaction of the health problem with certain Human Response systems. Anxiety and Dysfunctional grieving best fit with the Emotional human responses, while Family processes, altered, belongs to the Family Human Response System.

While this example is just one example of how nursing diagnoses might be organized for practice, it does seem a promising avenue to pursue. Much work would need to be undertaken to classify all of the phenomena into nursing diagnoses representing the intersection of human responses with health problems. Yet, for practicing nurses, the effort may be fruitful, as a usable and feasible, practice-friendly classification system is developed.

Another approach might be to specify nursing diagnoses likely to be found, given more abstract groupings of phenomena than "death of spouse" along the Actual and Potential Health Problem axis. Here, nursing diagnoses and health assessment strategies would be tailored along the six categories of the Human Response system axis, each interacting with a subcategory of an Actual or Potential Health Problem class. An example of how this approach might begin is illustrated in Figure 6 where the Developmental Life Change of Aging is linked to several human response system health behaviors. In actuality, the schema in Figure 6 served as the framework for Gale-Swanson's thesis (Gale-Swanson, 1986). Her results indicated areas of concern under the rubric of aging that point the way to development of groupings of phenomena or situations which have the potential to or are likely to occur.

Further work along the lines just described might eventually guide practitioners to development of computerized systems where nurses could indicate specific classification of Actual or Potential Health

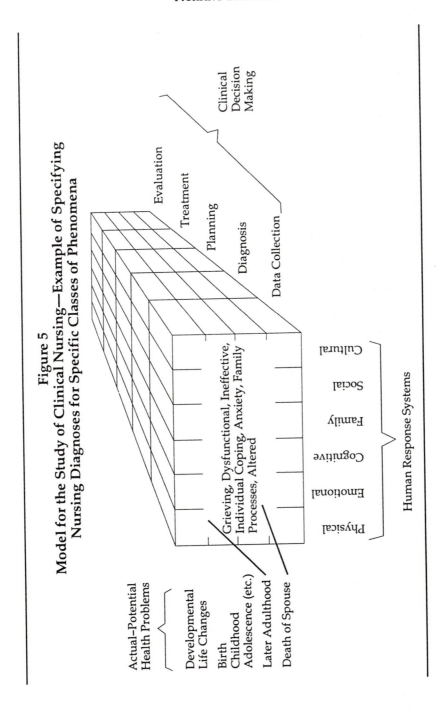

Figure 5
Model for the Study of Clinical Nursing—Example of Specifying
Nursing Diagnoses for Specific Classes of Phenomena

Figure 6
Gale-Swanson's Integrated Model for the Study of Health Behaviors of Elderly Individuals

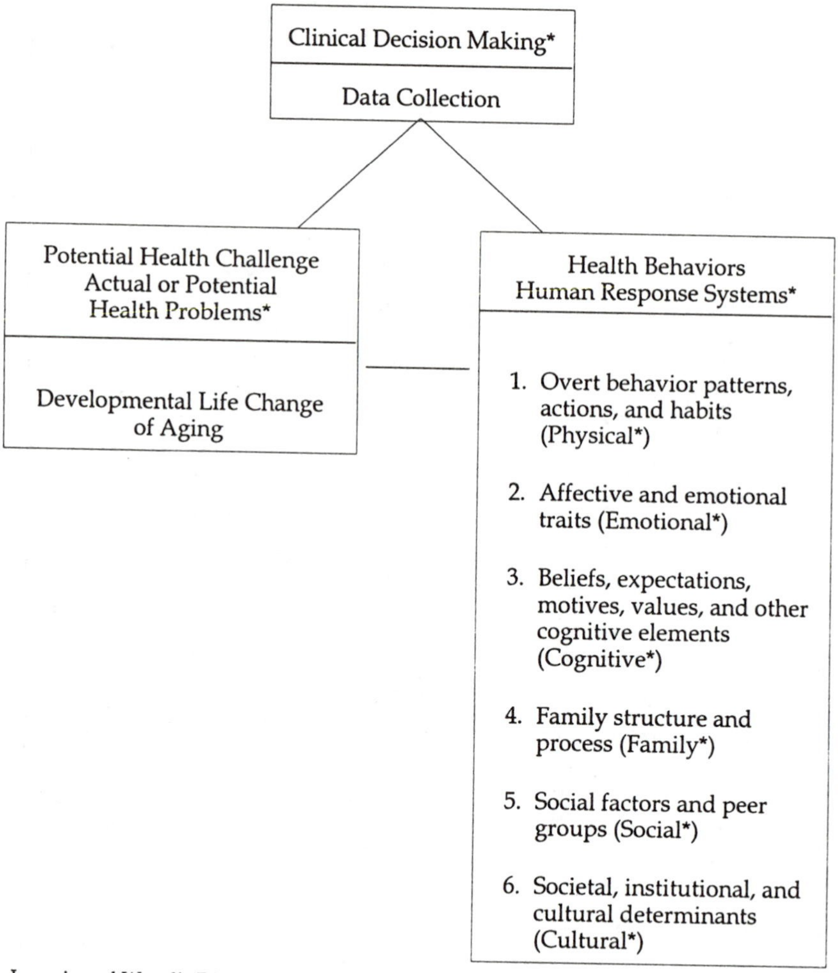

| Clinical Decision Making* |
| Data Collection |

| Potential Health Challenge Actual or Potential Health Problems* | Health Behaviors Human Response Systems* |
| Developmental Life Change of Aging | 1. Overt behavior patterns, actions, and habits (Physical*)

2. Affective and emotional traits (Emotional*)

3. Beliefs, expectations, motives, values, and other cognitive elements (Cognitive*)

4. Family structure and process (Family*)

5. Social factors and peer groups (Social*)

6. Societal, institutional, and cultural determinants (Cultural*) |

• Loomis and Wood's Dimensions.

Problem, then indicate Human Response categories. Logarithms could be constructed to alert the nurses to specific focal areas needing assessment. Assessment strategies shown through research to be worthwhile in each separate area could be stored in computer memory, to be offered as computer-generated suggestions for assessment strategies shown effective in either supporting or failing to support the actuality of certain nursing diagnoses, given certain pre-encounter and encounter data (Carnevali et al., 1984).

By the same token, nursing diagnoses which indicate or support health and wellness (Houldin, Saltstein, & Ganley, 1987) could also be included in any classification of nursing diagnostic phenomena using the Loomis/Wood Model. These diagnoses could also be incorporated in a computerized system as described above.

For example, the intersection of the Actual or Potential Health Problem axis category of Cultural and Environmental Stressors with the Human Response Systems of Cognitive, Social, or Family human response might, through empirical investigation, be found to indicate likelihood of several "wellness" diagnoses. This grouping of diagnoses conceivably might include "Effective crisis resolution" (Houldin et al., 1987, p. 171), "Effective social functioning" (p. 174), or "Effective family coping" (p. 179).

Either a computerized or noncomputerized system that incorporated wellness-based potential diagnoses would assist the nurse in assessing for strengths. Indication of positive characteristics could be utilitarian in nurses' efforts to support patients or clients toward desired outcomes in relation to any health problem. This approach would also serve to at least partially address one of the limitations of the Loomis/Wood Model, that of a focus on negative or problematic situations (see Chapter 1).

The preceding paragraphs described several potential uses of the Loomis/Wood Model for nurses' independent practice. Similar strategies could be instituted to begin to classify the phenomena associated with both interdependent and dependent nursing practice. One avenue available to accomplish this task would be for nurses to focus on, investigate, and begin to classify indicators of what Carpenito (1987) terms "collaborative problems" (p. 23). She defines collaborative problems as "the physiological complications that have resulted or may result from pathophysiological and treatment-related situations. Nurses monitor to detect their onset/status and collaborate with physicians for definitive treatment" (p. 24). Such efforts would go a long way toward clarifying the often confusing web of phenomena nurses are concerned with routinely.

THE LOOMIS/WOOD MODEL AS A
NURSING SERVICE ORGANIZER

The major effectiveness of any theoretical/conceptual framework for nursing lies in its usefulness for practicing nurses in their care of patients or clients. Another promising function of any nursing model, however, is its application as a means to organize a nursing service.

Stevens (1984) describes nursing service organizations where nursing theories, such as that of Roy (Mastal, Hammond, & Roberts, 1982), are used to organize not only the structure of the nursing department but also the functions of nurses within each unit.

Dream along as we tour a local hospital and health center which has hypothetically been organized using the Loomis/Wood Model. There are five major "centers" in our proposed nursing department. They are the Center for "Acute Health Deviations," the Center for "Chronic Health Deviations," the Center for "Developmental Life Changes," and of course, the "Cultural and Environmental Stressor Center." In addition, there is a "Home Health Care Center" which collaborates with all other centers. Within each center are units or sectors appropriate to classifications of Actual and Potential Health Problems encountered. For instance, the Center for "Acute Health Deviations" is composed of several inpatient units including Acute Illness, Acute Disease, the Trauma Sector, the Surgical Sector, Acute Psychiatric Sector, and an outpatient unit designed to assess and ameliorate acute episodes of illness, disease, or trauma not requiring hospitalization. Nurses in several of these sectors have joint appointments with the "Home Health Care Center," to which most patients having been hospitalized in the "Acute Health Deviation Center" are referred.

As we move along in our proposed facility, we come upon another major center, the "Center for Chronic Health Deviations." This center is composed of several units including traditional medical units, as well as a "Chronic Psychiatric Health Deviation Unit" and sectors focusing on treatment for classes of chronic health deviations such as the Cancer Care Sectors, the Joint and Bone Care Sector, and a special step-down unit, the Life-style Change Unit, which collaborates with many of the other "Chronic Health Deviation" Center Units. Here too, nurses have joint appointments with the "Home Health Care Center" to ensure continuity of care beyond hospitalization to home.

Out next stop is at the "Developmental Life Change Center," where we find units dedicated to assisting in life change transitions. Among the units here are the Maternal-Newborn Unit, the Childhood Development Unit where children are assisted with problematic aspects of adjustment and physical development, and the Hospice Unit, composed of both an inpatient and an outpatient hospice sector. Other outpatient services in this department target service to clients with other developmentally related aspects such as various parenthood transitions, women's developmental issues, men's developmental issues, phenomena associated with later life, and normative family transitions. As with all of the other centers, nurses from selected units such as the Maternal-Newborn Unit are jointly employed in the "Home Health Care Center."

Our final examination is of the "Cultural and Environmental Stressor" Center where we find an array of outpatient and community based clusters of activity focused on various stressors. One of these sectors is the occupational stressor sector where nurse consultants provide services to various businesses, manufacturing facilities, other organizations, and health center staff regarding healthful practices or conditions. These nurses also assist their organizational clients in developing prevention and health promotion policies and programs. Another sector in this center is the Family Catastrophic Stressor Sector, where family clinical nurse specialists work with families having experienced catastrophes that are "sudden, unexpected, frightening experiences for the individuals and families who survive them" (Figley & McCubbin, 1983, p. xix), with the goal of promoting adjustment and even growth within stressed families. At the end of our tour, we return to the Nursing Service Administrator's Office where he or she discusses with us other collaborative arrangements associated with these five centers. For instance, the local university's school of nursing is organized into four departments, the Acute Health Deviation Department, the Chronic Health Deviation Department, the Developmental Life Change Department, and the Cultural and Environmental Stressor Department. Nursing faculty at this school share joint appointments in the appropriate hospital center. The hospital nurses also frequently engage in activities jointly with the corresponding school of nursing department. This arrangement proves to be very beneficial to nursing students and to patients and clients.

In addition, many of the hospital nurses, as previously mentioned, share portions of their appointment with the hospital's "Home Health Care Center." This arrangement enhances the nursing care patients/ clients receive as they are discharged and after returning home. These nurses, many of whom also serve as cooperating clinicians with the local university school of nursing, are able to demonstrate to nursing students the real value of discharge planning, follow through, and continuity in the various aspects of health care. Moreover, this hospital employs the nursing diagnosis classification system based on the Loomis/Wood Model as previously described. All in all, our visit to this hypothetical hospital and health center has been a fascinating one. Loomis and Wood would be proud.

THE LOOMIS/WOOD MODEL IN
SPECIALTY NURSING PRACTICE

A third major purpose for a nursing conceptual framework in practice is as a framework for guiding specialty nursing practice. In this case, the conceptual model serves as an organizing structure with boundaries for the practice engaged in and for the work performed.

For example, a clinic-based nurse practitioner or a nurse entrepreneur engaged in independent practice (Vogel & Doleysh, 1988), focusing his or her efforts in the area of adult health, might delimit practice based on Loomis and Wood's categories of Actual and Potential Health Problems (Loomis & Wood, 1983). In this regard, some nurse practitioners or entrepreneurs may concentrate on "Chronic Health Deviations" with all of the associated human responses. Another practitioner, whose service is for mothers, father, and newborns, might converge his or her practice on the "Developmental Life Changes "of parenthood and birth. These are just two illustrations of how the model can be used to delimit practice organized creatively via the Loomis/Wood Model.

Another avenue for this type of model use could be in the practice of clinical nurse specialists. A family clinical nurse specialist's practice might center on the family unit's response to an acute health deviation. See, for example, Figure 7, where the family CNS "deliberately and consistently targeted nursing interventions at the level of the family unit" (Gilliss, 1991, p. 19). This approach would clearly exemplify specialty family nursing practice, different from the "family-as-context" approach (Gilliss, p. 19).

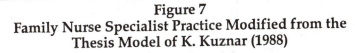

Figure 7
Family Nurse Specialist Practice Modified from the
Thesis Model of K. Kuznar (1988)

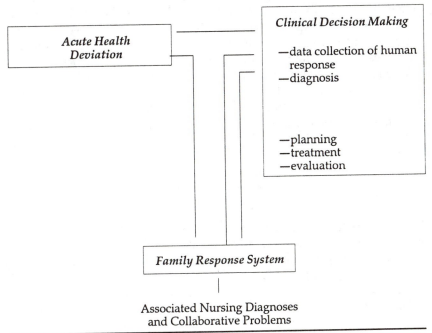

A broader and more circumspect arena for nursing practice bounded by the Loomis/Wood Model was developed by Paremski, Schams, and Yurkovich (1988). These clinical nurse specialists proposed the Loomis/Wood nursing conceptual framework as a model for CNS gerontological practice because, in their words, "Nursing care for the elderly has historically been based on the medical model, involving short-term treatment of acute illness. Since the health needs of this group are primarily chronic in nature, the medical model alone is insufficient to serve as a basis for care of the aged" (p. 15).

In their article, as in their practice, Paremski, Schams, and Yurkovich (1988), organize their nursing care primarily according to human responses to: (1) the developmental process of aging, (2) acute and chronic health deviations, and (3) cultural and environmental stressors. For example, in delimiting their gerontological practice concerning the Cultural and Environmental Stressors classification, these clinicians include the human responses in all six systems to ageism, relocation, potential poverty, cultural values, and limited financial resources.

These specialists also go on to explain how gerontological CNS's practice using all four of the prototypes of Loomis/Wood's Model (see Figure 4). According to Paremski, Schams, and Yurkovich (1988), "Loomis and Wood's Model for Clinical Nursing provides the flexibility necessary to diagnose and treat the variety of human responses elicited in the aged by an array of actual or potential health problems" (p. 17). Using the model in this way can ensure that specialty practice is indeed based on a nursing-developed definition of nursing fitting within the criteria developed by the American Nurses' Association for specialty nursing practice (ANA, 1980).

CONCLUSION

The possibilities for use of the Loomis/Wood Model in nursing practice are numerous. By using the Loomis/Wood Model, clinical nurses recognize the potential to "cure" by focusing on the human responses to actual and potential health problems. Loomis and Wood (1983) define cure as "evidenced by patient strategies and alternatives for dealing with stressors, smooth developmental and environmental transitions, and the absence of abnormal physical or emotional behavior" (p. 7). They further define cure as the "reversal or absence of aberrant human response" (p. 7) and as synonymous with care in some situations.

In addition, the model can serve as an organizer for nursing service or for specialty practice. Beyond these applications, other possibilities seem limitless. Creativity in this respect could be employed to develop even more fruitful functions for this legitimate and useful nursing conceptual framework. As ever more nurses begin to actually practice "nursing," this model has the potential of becoming the premiere nursing practice conceptual model.

REFERENCES

American Nurses' Association. (1980). *Nursing: A social policy statement.* Kansas City, MO: Author.

Carnevali, D., Mitchell, P., Woods, N., & Tanner, C. (1984). *Diagnostic reasoning in nursing.* Philadelphia: Lippincott.

Carpenito, L. J. (1987). *Nursing diagnosis: Application to clinical practice,* second edition. New York: Lippincott.

Carroll-Johnson, M. (1989). *Classification of nursing diagnoses: Proceedings of the Eighth Conference.* Philadelphia: Lippincott.

Figley, C. R., & McCubbin, H. (1983). *Stress and the family: Coping with catastrophe.* New York: Brunner/Mazel.

Gale-Swanson, E. (1986). *Health behaviors and the factors that influence health behaviors in an elderly population.* Unpublished Master's thesis, University of Wisconsin-Eau Claire.

Gebbie, K. (1982). Toward the theory development for nursing diagnoses classification. In M. Kim & D. Moritz (Eds.), *Classification of nursing diagnoses.* New York: McGraw-Hill.

Gilliss, C. L. (1991). Family nursing research, theory and practice. *Image: The Journal of Nursing Scholarship, 23*(1), 19–22.

Gordon, M. (1982a). *Nursing diagnosis: Process and application.* New York: McGraw-Hill.

Gordon, M. (1982b). Historical perspective: The national group for classification of nursing diagnoses. In M. Kim, D. Moritz (Eds.), *Classification of Nursing diagnoses.* New York: McGraw-Hill.

Houldin, A. D., Saltstein, S., & Ganley, K. (1987). *Nursing diagnoses for wellness.* Philadelphia: Lippincott.

Kritek, P. (1986). Development of a taxonomic structure for nursing diagnosis. In M. Hurley (Ed.), *Classification of nursing diagnoses: Proceedings of the Sixth Conference.* St. Louis: C. V. Mosby.

Kuznar, K. A. (1988). *The important needs of family members of critically ill patients.* Unpublished Master's thesis, University of Wisconsin-Eau Claire.

Loomis, M., & Wood, D. J. (1983). Cure: The potential outcome of nursing care. *Image: The Journal of Nursing Scholarship, 15*(1), 4–7.

Maas, M., Buckwalter, K. C., & Hardy, M. (1991). *Nursing diagnoses and interventions for the elderly.* Redwood City, CA: Addison-Wesley Nursing.

Mastal, M. F., Hammond, H., & Roberts, M. (1982). Theory into hospital practice: A pilot implementation. *Journal of Nursing Administration, 11*(6), 9–15.

Paremski, A., Schams, K. H., & Yurkovich, P. (1988). A conceptual model for CNS practice. *Journal of Gerontological Nursing, 14*(2), 14–18.

Roy, C. (1984). Framework for classification systems development: Progress and issues. In M. Kim, G. McFarland, & A. McLane (Eds.), *Classification of nursing diagnoses.* St. Louis: C. V. Mosby.

Stevens, B. J. (1984). *Nursing theory: Analysis, application, evaluation* (second edition). Boston: Little, Brown.

Vogel, G., & Doleysh, N. (1988). *Entrepreneuring: A nurse's guide to starting*

5

Models for the Next Century

Peggy L. Chinn

The task of evaluation and critique of a nursing model can be accomplished in many different ways. Several approaches to model and theory evaluation have been described in nursing's theoretically related literature (Chinn & Kramer, 1991; Fawcett, 1989). For the purposes of this critique, I have chosen to depart from the standard pedagogical approaches to evaluation and critique since this type of task can be accomplished by the well-informed student of nursing model and theory development. Rather, because the Loomis/Wood Model described in this book is identified as having considerable utility for the future of nursing education, research, and practice, I have chosen to critique the model based on a vision of what I anticipate the future to be by the year 2000.

My vision of the future, and the critique of the model that emerges from it, is based on two particular philosophic perspectives. One originates in nursing philosophy, the other in feminist philosophy. In an earlier article (Chinn, 1989) where I explore the connections between these two perspectives, I identified the fundamental tenet of nursing philosophy to be "health as wholeness," and that of feminism to be "the personal is political." Interestingly, while the Loomis/Wood Model is not designed specifically to address either of these tenets, in relating the evolution of Loomis and Wood's thinking, I have found these two tenets to have clearly influenced and shaped their thinking and development of the model. They clearly place their thinking in a epistemological tradition that compartmentalizes knowledge development into discrete units, yet the complexity of their model and the necessity to use multivariate techniques arises from the recognition that the whole is greater than the sum of the parts. Their use of the "ANA Social Policy Statement" definition of nursing, their inclusion of broad social and political concepts in various permutations of the model, and their application of the model to nursing research that addresses social and professional issues all speak to their awareness of places where the personal intersects with the political, and is political.

In the first section of this chapter, I will present a vision of the future in terms of (1) what is likely to change by the year 2000, (2) what is likely to remain stable through the early part of the next century, and (3) what is hanging in the balance. In the second section of this chapter, I will critique the Loomis/Wood Model in light of this vision of the future, including aspects of the model that hold promise for the future of the development of nursing and health care, and those aspects of the model that may not be adequate to that future.

PERSPECTIVES ON THE FUTURE

What Is Likely To Change By the Year 2000

In the next decade, four areas of drastic change are likely to appear: (1) an explosion of technology, (2) an evolution of devastating disease trajectories, (3) a drastic scarcity of resources in the face of increased demand for those resources, and (4) a dramatic increase in complexity in every arena of life.

Technology

By the year 2000, the technological milieu in which we live and work will look more like "Star Trek" than we can now imagine. The technological explosion that we have seen in the past decade is a hint of what we can anticipate in the future. In 1982, for example, the personal computer was just beginning to emerge on the market. FAX machines, cordless telephones, and autofocus cameras were almost unheard of. Voice mail and answering machines were only beginning to be used, and reluctantly by most people. Now, these are only a few of the technological "gadgets" that have become indispensable in the conduct of business and industry, as well as in the management of day-to-day living.

Those of us who work in high-tech medical environments are aware of the amazingly short half-life of the best and latest technology. By the year 2000, it will not be possible to work in a medical care institution without sophisticated computer skills; computers will be at every bedside, with ready access to not only the complete data base for the patient, but to entire libraries of information that could influence clinical decision making.

While the technological explosion is inevitable, there is not yet a clearly emerging sound basis for the formation of ethical solutions that high technology creates, and the decision-making processes that must accompany the application of technology (Pickerson, 1988; Henderson, 1985; Amos & Graves, 1990). As I will show later in this chapter, it is in this area that the future challenge rests for nurses.

Disease Trajectories

The basis for my grim forecast of devastating disease trajectories in the future is the fact of environmental destruction, waste, and pollution that human cultures and political systems are not yet equipped to recognize, much less address. As pliable and adaptable as the human organism is, I believe that we have ample evidence that we are reaching the limits of our ability to withstand the constant and devastating insults to health and well-being, and that we will continue to see increasingly tragic effects in terms of human health. Further, as resources become more scarce, more people will have less and less material support to engage in the kind of preventive care that will be required to withstand the effects of new disease trajectories.

Scarcity of Resources

We face a decade when we will see dramatic changes in the proportion of available resources available for the growing demand on those resources—financial resources, natural resources, and health care services. Additionally, the profit motive is destined to intensify, or there will need to be drastic reforms in the distribution of certain types of resources so that the profit motive no longer operates at its current expansive rate. Since the health care system in the United States has been long entrenched in a capitalist structure where profit is the primary motive that directs the use and distribution of resources, and in which huge profits are still made at untold cost to human lives, it will take an incredible effort to shift to a system where profit is not the primary motivation.

Increasing Complexity

Complexity has already become a familiar way of life for many, but complexity will increasingly become a dominant theme in human experience. The technology explosion contributes to the foreseen increase in complexity, particularly with respect to making possible the information explosion that accompanies it. But technology alone, and the information explosion that goes with it, will not account for the phenomenon I am addressing. Increasing complexity will emerge in part by the practical necessity to take into account more people and hence more points of view; a necessity, if you will, to synthesize more and more "stuff" into less and less time and space. As people of the world become more literate and westernized, their voices will demand a greater forum for recognition, for sharing in the shrinking of world resources, and for gaining the power of choice in what solutions are created to deal with *global* problems. Hence, complexity arises from emerging political, philosophic, social, environmental, and cultural diversity that must merge if we are all to survive on this planet.

In all world cultures, provisions for health and well-being and for treatment of disease will also become exceedingly complex. The successes and the failures of western allopathic medicine and nursing will become increasingly evident as the philosophies and practices of other healing modalities worldwide can no longer be ignored. As in many other arenas of life, no longer will it be possible to assume that there is any *one* way to do something, nor that only one type of practitioner can do it.

What Is Likely to Not Change

Just as there are things that can reasonably be predicted to change, there are also things that can reasonably be predicted to not change, or to remain stable—at least for the next eight to ten years unless there is a major planetary disaster (i.e., nuclear war) that catapults Earth cultures into something entirely different. The four areas that are likely to not change are: (1) the context of worldwide patriarchal dominance, (2) oppression as a persistent pattern of relationship between groups of people, (3) a human demand for freedom and quality of life, and (4) a human yearning for connection and meaning in relationships with others.

Patriarchal Dominance

Patriarchal dominance refers to a system of thinking that has its roots in the assumption that whatever is assigned "male" characteristics is superior to that which is assigned "female" characteristics. It does not necessarily refer to individuals who are female or male. More fundamentally, it refers to seeing people, objects, behaviors, even nature (i.e., the moon, sun, earth, sky) as imbued with gender traits, and those objects, behaviors, and traits that are seen as male as better, more valuable, to be noticed, the standard of measure, and so forth (Chinn & Wheeler, 1985).

In the health care system, what emerges from patriarchal dominance on the surface is the dominance of a predominantly male profession over a profession that is predominantly female. However, even if the distribution of men and women in nursing or medicine were to shift, the general attitude that one is worth more than the other, or that one gains notices over the other, or that one gains recognition of a credibility greater than the other, will not readily shift, because one type of work is viewed as essentially male in character and the other as essentially female in character.

Patriarchal dominance is not likely to change because it is embedded in all human cultures worldwide for most of recorded history. In western culture, even though we have made significant gains with respect to "equal rights" for women, the tendency to assign gender-specific valence to people, objects, events, and processes remains firmly planted in every indicator of culture and experience. For example, westerners typically impose an essential "female-male" interpretation on the Chinese concepts of "yin and yang," erroneously viewing these as "male and female." While this is symptomatic of the cultural tendency to "genderize," it is more fundamentally symptomatic of the patriarchal habit of thinking that polarizes, dichotomizes, overly simplifies, categorizes, and pigeonholes almost everything and anything. In addition, each end of a dichotomous spectrum is automatically assigned certain value traits. In this context, we find it unthinkable that one thing can be equal to another, or simply different, or even parts of a large whole.

Oppression

While oppression as a pattern of relationships between groups of people is closely related to the pattern of patriarchal dominance, patriarchal dominance alone cannot account for the worldwide tendency of groups of people within and between cultures to engage in a pattern of dominance and submission when relating with one another. Like patriarchal dominance, patterns of oppressive relationships are now embedded in human relations, and as such they are not likely to change easily or quickly (Freire, 1970).

The control of knowledge is the most powerful tool that sustains oppressive relationships. It is true that the burgeoning technological advances and the information explosion may undermine oppressive relationships. However, what "counts" as legitimate information and as legitimate "technology" is fundamentally defined by the value system of those who have the power and the influence to prescribe *legitimate* values. Knowledge is fundamentally controlled by the value system that underlies it and the value system that defines what to count as worthwhile and good for whom. In nursing, as long as we view one type of knowledge (such as knowledge associated with allopathic medicine) as more valuable than other types of knowledge (such as knowledge of human caring or of alternative healing modalities), we will continue to grant legitimacy to a system of oppression. We reflect the oppressive nature of relationships between groups of health care providers when involved in internal debates about what knowledge and skills "belong" to which sub-group of nurses, thus sustaining a debilitating and non-productive pattern for nursing's future by many divisive internal relationships between one another.

Desire for Freedom and Quality of Life

Ironically, theories of oppression also enlighten another circumstance that will not change in the foreseeable future—the human yearning for freedom from oppression and for a better quality of life. Just as oppressive relationships between people have a history as long as recorded memory, so does the human effort to gain freedom from oppression and injustice and to achieve a better quality of life. People continue to seek freedom from political oppression of the state, people of color seek freedom from systematic racism and related forms of oppression, and women as a "class" for centuries have written and spoken of their struggles for individual and collective freedom and quality of life and how this has been denied them through patriarchal control.

Nurses have spoken and written of the right to control nursing practice since Florence Nightingale first envisioned an autonomous nursing profession. Like the larger social and political movements for freedom, nurses' efforts to gain autonomy are inevitably linked to a vision of quality of care and, in turn, a quality of life for the caregiver and for the care recipient.

Connection and Meaning in Relationships with Others

Human yearning for connection and meaning in relationships with others is a steady undercurrent that accounts for far more than appears on first view. Superficially, many efforts toward human liberation seem to be seeking freedom from oppression. Many such efforts are equally motivated by a yearning for meaningful connections that are missing in oppressive relationships. For example, when nurses contemplate and speak about seeking "autonomy" in practice, nurses are motivated by that yearning, at least in part. As heard by others as themselves, nurses seem to express here a yearning for freedom from the unreasonable constraints that are placed on nursing practice by groups other than nursing or individuals other than nurses. In my experience, what nurses usually mean, and often take one another to mean, is that nurses are seeking a quality of relationship that can only exist when nurses "count" themselves as fully qualified, capable individuals—capable of making judgments, decisions, and of knowing when and how to work with others. In this sense, what nurses are really seeking is not so much freedom (although that certainly is an issue in many cases) as it is a *quality of connection* with everyone involved in practice situations that endows all with abilities to exercise human skill, judgment, and interaction.

WHAT IS HANGING IN THE BALANCE

As we approach the next century, there are three areas that are critical to the future of nursing and health care and that are hanging in the balance: (1) the ethical basis for making decisions, (2) the value basis for health and healing knowledge and practice, and (3) the necessity of shifting from essential individualism to essential collectivism and valuing of diversity.

The Ethical Basis for Making Decisions

In the past, the predominant ethic on which decisions have been made include an ethic of justice, or rights, and responsibilities. This ethic is incumbent in patriarchal thinking, and it will continue to enter into ethical deliberations. However, as Noddings (1989) has so clearly explained, this standpoint is no longer adequate by itself. An ethic based on and that arises from human relationships, or an ethic of caring and connection, brings into nursing's realm of understanding a totally new view of what is possible. A growing library of nursing literature that supports and enlightens alternative bases for ethical decision making, bringing nurses to the cutting edge of what is possible in the future, is one significant result of that new view.

The Value Basis for Health and Healing Knowledge and Practice

As quality of life grows increasingly threatened, and the limitations of allopathic medicine become increasingly apparent, and assuming that all individuals will continue to seek a better quality of life and health, then we, as nurses, are at a critical crossroads in making value judgments as to "right," "effective," and "good" ways to do so. Likewise, we are at a critical crossroads for making sound judgments as to how health and healing are to be defined.

If nurses are to influence the directions of health and healing in the future, nurses can no longer ignore alternative healing modalities. Nurses can no longer devalue the knowledge that is needed to practice those modalities. Nurses cannot rely on the profit-motivated health care system as known for the past several decades to ensure nurses a "place" in a century that is to be plagued by devastating disease trajectories and by scarce resources. Nurses can choose to see increasing complexity as an opportunity, and choose to embrace that complexity in every aspect of practice. Intuition, the art of nursing, esthetics knowledge, personal knowledge, knowledge of relationships, knowledge of "paranormal" phenomena, and unlimited other types of knowledge will become increasingly necessary. Of course, many of the "knowledges" that have been denied to nurses are those associated with femaleness in a patriarchal system, and with submissiveness in a dominant-submissive oppressive relationship. If nurses are to swing the balance where knowledge is concerned, our first challenge is to begin to value that which we have learned to devalue as knowledge.

The Possibility for Collectivism and Valuing Diversity

Fundamental to our ability to value what nurses have learned to devalue, and to integrate complexity into nursing practice, will be our ability to shift from an essential orientation of individualism to an essential orientation of collectivity. Nursing's debates about entry into practice, defining "roles" of various types of practitioners, or nursing's efforts to "simplify" nursing credentialing stems from what we have been taught to value in terms of "status" in a hierarchal system of health care that emphasizes individuality, and serves primarily to divide nurses from one another—a powerful tool to sustain oppressive relationships.

When nurses move toward recognizing the inherent value of our diversity and bring together various perspectives, skills, and talents in order to meet the increasing and complex needs of the people nurses serve, then nurses will begin to see ways in which nurses can work effectively together as nurses move toward the next century.

CRITIQUE OF THE LOOMIS/WOOD MODEL

When viewed in light of projections and possibilities for the future, the Loomis/Wood Model reveals promise and limitations. The promise for the future use of the model rests fundamentally in its flexibility; the limitations rest in the fact that certain understanding and insight that is needed for the future is that for which the model is not designed.

Potential Structures for Data Bases

A major strength of the Loomis/Wood Model is the endless possibilities for organization and integration of information into a cohesive and useable whole. The technological explosion will make the design of data bases increasingly accessible to more and more "users." Further, as these data bases become more accessible, the possibilities for calculating and integrating data into relationships derived from mathematical principles and statistics is endless. The model provides a structure that can give conceptual meaning to the selection of data; it also provides a structure that gives conceptual meaning to the relationships between and among data. Although the model does not ensure conceptual integrity of data or of relationships, it does provide an initial grounding in concepts that are central to nursing, and it acknowledges the fundamental commitment in nursing to recognizing important relationships among variables that might otherwise be seen as disconnected. As Loomis and Wood acknowledge, their model is not a tool for discerning the whole in the sense that might be philosophically desirable in nursing, but it does require integration of relationships among variables in a way that is likely to be useful for many circumstances in the foreseeable future. The technological explosion of the future will make possible sophisticated treatment of the types of relationships that are implied in the model.

Broad Spectrum of Abstraction Related to Health and Illness

The Loomis/Wood Model incorporates a broad spectrum of abstraction related to health and illness. As disease trajectories worsen and affect more people, and as the relationships between environmental and social issues and health/illness phenomena become more evident, a model that integrates many possible variables at all levels of abstraction will become increasingly useful. Consistent with nursing's historical commitment to wellness, while at the same time responding to the realities of disease and illness, this model makes it possible to account for a range of possibilities in health and illness processes.

The strength of the model in not prescribing what these levels of abstraction are also signifies its limitation. While nurses can insert whatever range of abstraction is well suited to the specific situation, the model does not prompt conceptualizations of health and illness, or of social, environmental, or political processes that move beyond traditional conceptualizations. However, as nurses begin to move toward new insights concerning health and illness, and healing processes inherent in nursing, new conceptualizations can be used.

Utility and Efficacy

As resources become increasingly scarce and as demand for the use of resources becomes greater, the ability to document and to demonstrate the utility and efficacy of nursing care is imperative. The Loomis/Wood Model provides a framework within which this can be accomplished. Even more important, the model "demands" that variables central to nursing's concerns be accounted for in the study of efficacy or outcome. If nursing's concerns are to be considered in decisions about resource utilization in the future, it will be incumbent upon nurse practitioners and researchers to define the terms upon which efficacy is to be conceived and the data upon which judgments will be built. The Loomis/Wood Model points the way to inclusion of at least a broad spectrum of human responses, the full range of actual and potential health-related processes, and the essential processes of nursing judgment and action.

Potential for Parsimonious Treatment of Data

The Loomis/Wood Model provides a conceptually accessible and general framework for organizing highly complex data. As Werner

points out, one reason the Loomis/Wood Model "works" in the clinical setting better than other methods of classification of nursing
diagnoses is its easily understood and simple structure for classification. In a future of increasing complexity, a framework that makes it
possible to integrate more and more into a parsimonious whole will
be extremely valuable. Further, the flexibility of the model to incorporate changing data, and to tailor that data input with respect to a
particular situation, speaks to the potential for parsimonious treatment of data that is inherent in the model.

The danger with respect to integration of complex data is that
uniqueness, qualitatively important variation, or nuances or meaning
are easily lost. In this light, the Loomis/Wood Model will not be well
suited in situations where uniqueness and nuance of meaning are of
primary concern. However, as more sophisticated possibilities evolve
for treatment of numeric data and where phenomena can be
"translated" into numerical meaning effectively, it will become more
possible to reveal permutations of meaning in that data.

Limitations of Classification

In any model that requires classification of data or reduction of
phenomena to increasingly larger "classes" of abstraction, another
danger remains: errors of conceptual judgment can be made. In
addition, once a judgment is made to "classify" something in a particular way, that something may become something it is not. For
example, if a nurse views a human response as "coping," but the
person experiencing the situation does not see it this way, the nurse
may have made an "error" in judgment, or at least imposed a view that
is not well suited to the situation. A model that prompts classification
and diagnosis can also facilitate and sustain paternalistic relationships
that are grounded in patriarchal dominance.

Conceptual clarity on the part of nurses who use the model can
assist to overcome this limitation. However, conceptual clarity alone
will not suffice to ensure that the limitations of classification are
sufficiently addressed. Ethical issues, particularly with respect to "*who
gets to decide*" will be critical in the future. Clarity with respect to the
basis of ethical decision making, and shifting to an ethic of caring and
relationship rather than a strict ethic of justice, will be fundamental in
moving away from patriarchal dominance and paternalism in the
future.

Opportunity for and Limitations of Defining Knowledge

The Loomis/Wood Model provides a very broad structure for defining the type of knowledge that is "included," and that structure itself provides a value statement for the profession. The act of identifying what "counts" as admissible knowledge is a powerful tool that can be used to replicate and sustain oppressive forms of relationship.

Because the model structure for identifying what counts as knowledge is very broad, the limits are not easily discerned. The limits lie in the fact that this is not a model for resistance to the dominant paradigm; it provides structure for concepts that rest clearly within the dominant paradigm. As conceptualizations of health and illness phenomena emerge and paradigm shifts occur over the coming decade, the limitations of the model with respect to what is "admissible" may become more clear.

One limitation is that the model implies a reliance on observable and measurable data. In practice contexts where accountability and efficacy must be demonstrated, this is a strength. In practice contexts where experiential meaning or ethical dilemmas prevail, this is a limitation. Being aware of these strengths and limitations, it will be possible to make better informed judgments concerning the application and utility of the model.

Ethics, Values, Meaning, and Quality

Values and meaning are human ideas that pervade all human experiences. What typically counts as "science" has not been responsive to these human concerns; the philosophic tradition from which the Loomis/Wood Model emerged is this tradition of "science." Like science itself, the Loomis/Wood Model can be used as a tool to reveal ethics, values, meaning, and quality. Likewise, the philosophic and spiritual bases that undergird the concepts that are selected for the model might create subtle shifts in the model itself, just as they are creating shifts in the conceptions and processes of science. Just as we now speak of "human science" to signify conceptions and processes that move beyond the traditional scientific model, we might also begin to see potential for alternative conceptions and processes possible within the Loomis/Wood Model. It is a model that is sufficiently robust for this possibility to emerge.

CONCLUSION

In summary, the Loomis/Wood Model offers potential to influence what hangs in the balance for the future. It is a model that encompasses conceptual and ideological diversity. It is a model that encourages the use of empirical data applied within a framework of nursing's conceptual and ethical tradition. It is a model that can incorporate rapidly changing demands for more and sometimes different information. It does not prescribe; rather, it encourages contextual and situationally relevant choice on the part of the user. In my view, these are the types of features that will be critical for the next century.

REFERENCES

Amos, L. K., & Graves, J. R. (1990). Knowledge technology: costs, benefits, ethical considerations. In J. C. McCloskey & H. K. Grace (Eds.), *Current issues in nursing*. St. Louis: C. V. Mosby, 592–600.

Chinn, P. (1989). Nursing patterns of knowing and feminist thought. *Nursing and Health Care, 19*(2), 71–75.

Chinn, P., & Kramer, M. (1991). *Theory and nursing: A systematic approach*. St. Louis: C. V. Mosby.

Chinn, P., & Wheeler, C. (1985). *Nursing Outlook, 33*(2), 74–77.

Dickerson, J. (1988, June). Ethical problems in the advancement of medical technology. *Journal of the Royal Society of Health, 108*(3), 86–89.

Fawcett, J. (1989). *Analysis and evaluation of conceptual models in nursing (2nd ed.)*. Norwalk, CT: Appleton & Lange.

Freire, P. (1970). *Pedagogy of the oppressed*. New York: The Seabury Press.

Fry, S. (1989). Toward a theory of nursing ethics. *Advances in Nursing Science, 11*(2), 9–22.

Henderson, V. (1985, summer). The essence of nursing in high technology, *Nursing Administration Quarterly, 9*(4), 1–9.

Noddings, N. (1989). *Women and evil*. Berkeley: University of California Press.

Appendix

Cure: The Potential Outcome
of Nursing Care

Maxine E. Loomis
D. Jean Wood

ABSTRACT

The recent Social Policy Statement of the American Nurses' Association (1980) has advanced a definition of nursing as "the diagnosis and treatment of human responses to actual or potential health problems." This definition has legitimized efforts of the last decade to develop a system of nursing diagnosis and should provide the impetus

The authors wish to acknowledge the stimulation of Carol Dittamble, Helen Grace, and the U. of Illinois at Chicago, College of Nursing faculty in refining these ideas.

Loomis, M.E., & Wood, D.J. (1983, winter). Cure: The potential outcome of nursing care. *Image, The Journal of Nursing Scholarship, 25,*(1), 4–7.

125

*for subsequent development of nursing treatment interventions.
Barnard (1982) has proposed a model for linking the phenomenon of
concern to nursing with the human responses present in the maternal-
child nursing situation. Other specialty models are likely to follow.*

In this article we present the possibility that in the diagnosis and
treatment of human responses, nurses are capable of curing the actual
or potential health problem. The most recent definition of nursing has
opened up exploration of the interactions among human response
systems and actual or potential health problems. Clinicians, researchers, and theoreticians are now in a position to reconceptualize
nursing's impact on health and health problems.

DEVELOPMENT OF THE MODEL

Taken literally, the ANA definition implies a set of linear relationships.
When an actual or potential health problem invades or "comes over"
patients they respond from one or several human response systems;
the nurse diagnoses and treats the response(s). Unfortunately, clinical
practice is not that simple. In reality, any factor in the equation can
affect any other. A human response called "stress" might be related to
the onset of an acute illness episode. Conversely, the presence of a
chronic health deviation might complicate a developmental life
change, as in the case of an adolescent with cystic fibrosis. It is even
possible that the nursing treatment could induce or, at least increase
stress, illness, or health problems. What is required is a multivariate
model in which all human response systems interact with all actual or
potential human health problems as well as with the clinical decision-
making process.

The model in Figure 1 provides a schematic representation of the
possible relationships among actual or potential health problems,
human response systems, and clinical nursing decision making.*
What is proposed is a schema for categorizing actual or potential
health problems into (a) developmental life changes, (b) acute
health deviations, (c) chronic health deviations, and (d) culturally
and environmentally-induced stressors. With the presence of at least
one of these four factors, there is no actual or potential health
problem.

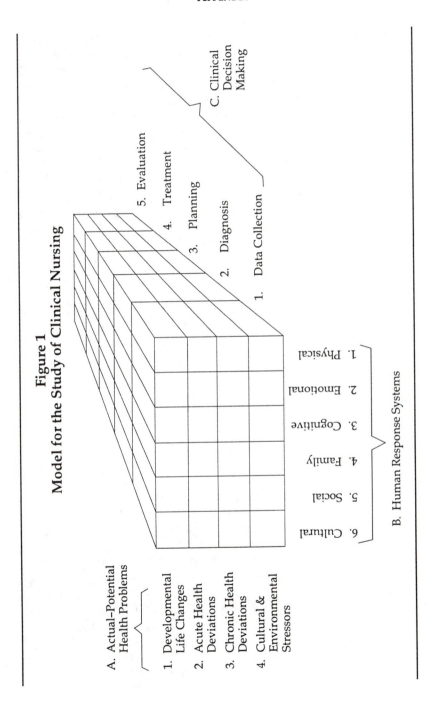

Figure 1
Model for the Study of Clinical Nursing

We propose that there are six human response systems in which a person can respond to actual or potential health problems: (a) physical, (b) emotional, (c) cognitive, (d) family, (e) social, and (f) cultural. It is possible, even probable, that more than one response system can be engaged in dealing with actual or potential health problems. For example, an acute illness episode may invoke physical, emotional, cognitive, and family system responses. Certain cultural or environmental stressors will call for family and social responses; while others may activate physical and cultural adjustments.

Clinical decision making as proposed in this model follows the familiar problem-solving steps of the nursing process. The goal of the process is straightforward: The diagnosis and treatment of human responses to actual or potential health problems. Within the process, Henderson's (1961) definition of nursing is still appropriate.

> . . . to assist the individual, sick or well, in the performance of those activities contributing to health or its recovery (or to a peaceful death) that he would perform unaided if he had the necessary strength, will or knowledge. And to do this in such a way as to help him gain independence as rapidly as possibly.

CLINICAL UTILITY

The possible interaction effects among human response systems, actual and potential health problems, and clinical decision making as outlined in the above model present nurses with many exciting possibilities for clinical practice, research, and theory development.

The notion that human response systems interact with and influence states of health has been popularized by authors such as Benson (1979), Brown (1975), Cousins (1979), Pelletier (1977), and Simonton and Simonton (1978). Scientific support for the proposition that health status responds to human volitional control comes from studies that demonstrate that certain brain-wave patterns can be detected and self-regulated (Kamiya, 1969), that some peripheral vascular responses can be controlled (Lynch & Shuri, 1978), and that particular visceral functions can be operantly conditioned (Roberts, 1978). The term "self-regulation" refers to the process of control of psychophysiologic states, a process facilitated by the focusing of attention (Green & Green, 1977). Existing data about self-regulation have been derived mainly from biofeedback studies involving both outpatients or healthy volunteers. In these studies, one or another strategy—instrumented biofeedback or noninstrumented biofeedback—for focusing attention has been used with subjects to induce self-regulatory responses (Kamiya, Barber, Miller, Shapiro, & Stoyva, 1977; Schwartz & Shapiro, 1976–1978).

Recent developments in the clinical application of biofeedback, visualization, systematic relaxation, cognitive restructuring, and related techniques have also provided support for the proposition that health status is subject to self-regulatory control (Kamiya et al., 1977; Meichenbaum, 1977; Schwartz, 1976; Shapiro, 1978). In particular, research in the area of biofeedback has contributed to the development of what is known as the "Psychophysiological principle." According to Green and Green (1977) this principle states:

Every change in the physiological state is accompanied by an appropriate change in the mental-emotional state, conscious or unconscious, and conversely, every change in the mental-emotional state, conscious or unconscious is accompanied by an appropriate change in the physiological state (p. 33)

This principle suggests that human self-regulatory processes are always in operation and that they may be more or less adequate to the stimuli to which the person is responding. It is when the self-regulatory response is inadequate or dysfunctional that there is need for professional assistance.

The following examples of the utility of the model for the study of clinical nursing are organized by four prototypes of health care situations. These are situations in which:

1. Health problems precede human responses.
2. Human responses precede health problems.
3. Health problems are defined by human responses.
4. Health problems interact with human responses.

Each health care situation will be discussed in terms of the clinical nursing model, examples will be provided, and treatment and cure will be discussed.

Health Problems Precede Human Responses

This category is perhaps the best prototype of the medical model role in action. Some disease or invasive organism overcomes the patient—hepatitis, herpes, influenza, or physical injury caused by an accident—and the episode is regarded as an acute health deviation. Primary treatment efforts are mobilized either to deter the invasive organism or to repair the damage caused by trauma. Medical and nursing interventions are directed to correcting physiologic damage and preventing additional physical complications. The physical human response system is of primary concern; emotional, cognitive, and family response systems are of secondary concern.

For example, a 49-year-old father and his 12-year-old daughter are brought to the Emergency Room following a car accident. His initial treatment requires surgery to close a sucking chest wound, and she requires orthopedic attention for arm and leg fractures. Nursing interventions for the first 48 hours for both patients will focus primarily on their physiologic human responses to their acute health deviations. Pain, fluids and electrolytes, and cardiovascular indicies of human responses to the trauma will all be monitored and adjusted. As father and daughter recover physically, nursing attention will gradually shift to the emotional impact of the accident and its effect on the patients' relationship with each other as well as the family structure. In a first-rate hospital with sensitive nursing staff the mother and siblings would be receiving simultaneous help with their emotional and cognitive responses to the accident while the identified patients were recovering from their acute physical crises. Nurses would be available to help them plan to cope with the needs of all family members during the period of treatment and recovery.

In situations where health problems precede human responses, cure has two foci. The initial focus of medical and nursing diagnosis and treatment is on the actual health problem (i.e., deterrence of the invasive organism or repair of the actual physical damage). Physiologic response systems are of primary importance, with emotional, cognitive, family and social response systems emphasized to assist patients and their support systems in coping with the acute health deviation. Cure is usually defined by (a) readjustment of the temporary physiologic/physical imbalance, and (b) patient and support system coping with the acute health deviation. Nurses are collaborators with physicians in the first aspect of cure and are collaborators with the patient and his/her support system in the second aspect of cure.

Human Responses Precede Health Problems

Developmental life changes such as puberty, marriage, pregnancy, divorce, and retirement can precipitate health care problems. For example, pregnancy is a significant life event that can trigger a variety of health problems for the unprepared. Prenatal visits provide physicians and nurses with the opportunity to monitor response systems and to provide necessary information and counsel regarding such factors as diet and exercise so that health problems do not occur. Lamaze classes in particular are designed to prevent negative outcomes through assisting couples to learn how to regulate response systems during labor and delivery.

Cultural and environmental stressors can play a significant role in potentiating health care problems. The current economic recession concerns nurses as a serious problem of health care as well as a social problem. For example, we now have epidemiologic proof that unemployment can proceed deaths by suicide and cardiovascular disease; there is also an increase in spouse and child abuse. The situation of child abuse poses unique problems for nurses and other health care workers because the child's health problem can only be palliatively treated without directly confronting the likelihood that the primary health problem may be the parents' response to stress. Reporting incidents of child abuse may or may not assist the parents to reassess their situation and alter their responses to stress.

The focus of treatment in these situations is on the human responses to developmental life changes and cultural and environmental life stressors. Nurses can help patients to adapt to life changes and remove or adjust to stressors. If an actual health problem has already developed, nurses give their attention to reversing existing mental or physical damage and preventing further disability. In the case of child abuse, nurses must attend to the immediate physical needs of the child and help the parents to secure adequate treatment for the child. Concurrently, nurses can help the parents to develop strategies and alternatives for dealing with the work, marital, and/or environmental stressors that have precipitated their abusive behavior.

By helping patients deal with their human responses to developmental or environmental stressors, nurses can prevent some potential health care problems. "Cure" is evidenced by smooth developmental and environmental transitions and the absence of abnormal physical or emotional behavior. Nurses are clearly prepared to assist patients with these human responses that precede actual or potential health care problems.

Health Problems Are Defined by Human Responses

The third category of health care situations are those in which the actual or potential health problems are defined by the human responses associated with them. "Fever of unknown origin" is a medical diagnosis defined by symptoms minus evidence of invasive organisms. Many psychiatric diagnoses fall into this same category

The third edition of the *Diagnostic and Statistical Manual* of the American Psychiatric Association (1980) presents a set of diagnostic categories based on specific configurations of symptoms or behaviors that are human responses. For example, Generalized Anxiety Disorder is "manifested by symptoms from three of the following four categories: (1) motor tension, (2) autonomic hyperactivity, (3) apprehensive expectation, (4) vigilance and scanning" (pp. 134–135). An adult who manifests this anxious mood continuously for at least one month when the problem is not attributable to another mental disorder would be diagnosed as having a generalized anxiety disorder.

In this case the nursing diagnosis would be the same as the medical diagnosis, given that the health problem is defined by the human response. Nursing treatment would focus on strategies for decreasing motor tension, decreasing autonomic hyperactivity, decreasing apprehensive expectations, and decreasing vigilance and scanning. Cure would be defined and documented in terms of physiologic, emotional, cognitive, and social relaxation—all within the scope of nursing practice. While there may be a need for intermittent biochemical intervention (psychotropic drugs to provide relief during acute episodes), cure can be found in correction of the human responses to anxiety-producing situations. The primary focus of diagnosis and treatment in this category is on the human response systems, with which nurses are most familiar and adept.

Health Problems Interact with Human Responses

Chronic health deviations such as adult-onset diabetes or chronic respiratory disease provide example of health problems that require equal attention to the health problem *and* the human response. Without the active cooperation of the patient, these health problems cannot be effectively treated. In addition to their medical regimens, these conditions usually require changes in life-style. Nurses might find it a challenge to assist these patients to include creatively their medical regimens into their definitions of themselves as spouses, employees, parents, or children. With chronic health care problems in particular it is essential that patients be willing to attend to internal cues about their health state and accept responsibility for negotiating modifications either in their activities or in their medical regimen. Some patients are not willing or able to do this and their health problem progresses despite treatment. Other patients improve without treatment because they voluntarily make radical changes in their life-style to self-regulate their health deviation. Most of these patients require the assistance of nurses and physicians to help them learn to attend to bodily cues and negotiate environmental demands.

Three patients exemplify the interaction between chronic health deviations and human response systems:

- The first is a 50-year old high school coach and math teacher with COPD who refused to acknowledge his changing health status, continued smoking, avoided medical or nursing treatment, and had to resign himself to the life of an invalid within seven years of his initial diagnosis.

- The second is a 45-year-old university professor who took her allergic asthma diagnosis as a challenge. She agreed to an initial course of bronchodilators to relieve her acute respiratory distress, began a program of systematic relaxation, initiated a progressive program of exercise and jogging, and altered her work environment to eliminate unnecessary stress. When she decided to reduce and gradually eliminate her medication, she was well on her way to the relatively symptom-free life she now enjoys fifteen years later. She still has the potential for respiratory problems, but she monitors her stress, exercise, and allergens carefully so as not to exacerbate her condition.

- The third patient is a 70-year-old woman diagnosed with inoperable lung cancer, who was told that she had only six months to live. Five years later she died comfortably with her extended family and friends caring for her in her home. She and her oldest son had managed her care, calling on personal friends and health care professional when necessary. Her latest months were managed, pain-free with the assistance of a hospice nurse.

For each of these patients, the interaction between their chronic health deviation and their human response systems was obvious and individual. They dealt with their health deviations in a way that fit with their respective life-styles. The challenge for the health care professionals—nurses in particular—in these cases was to adjust their clinical prescriptions to accommodate the self-regulatory processes of each individual. In the first case the patient fought the health care system, the system fought him, and they are now dependent on each other. In the second case, the patient collaborated with the health care system and is doing fine. In the third case, the patient and her support system contracted with the health care system for what she needed, and she died the way she chose.

"Cure" in each of these cases is measured by the effective management of the chronic health deviation with minimal disruption to the person's personal, professional, and social functioning. The focus of nursing diagnosis and treatment is on patients' self-regulation of the human responses that interact with their health problems. Nursing treatment may result in the reversal of a chronic disease process. In most cases effective nursing treatment will facilitate the ongoing management of what could be a debilitating process.

SUMMARY

Nursing care can cure. In this article we have attempted to expand the ANA definition of nursing into a model of clinical nursing and apply that model to four prototypes of actual or potential health problems. We have presented the possibility that when actual health problems proceed human responses, nurses collaborate with physicians in treating the physiological response to the acute health problem and collaborate with the patient and his/her support system in treating the emotional, cognitive, family, and social responses.

When human responses precede health problems, nurses are in a position to prevent potential health care problems by helping patients deal with their responses to developmental and/or environmental stressors. "Cure" is evidenced by patient strategies and alternatives for dealing with stressors, smooth developmental and environmental transitions, and the absence of abnormal physical or emotional behavior.

When health problems are defined by human responses, the nursing diagnosis is the same as the medical diagnosis. "Cure" is defined as the reversal or absence of aberrant human responses, and these are clearly the domain of nursing practice.

When health problems are interactive with human response systems "care" and "cure" may be synonymous. Care and cure involve effective mediation among medical treatment, health deviations, and life-styles. When health problems are interactive with human response systems nurses collaborate with physicians in treating the health deviation but are most active with patients and their support systems. The focus of nursing diagnosis and treatment is on patient and support system self-regulation of the human responses that interact with their health problems.

Nurses can cure people by helping them treat and cure themselves. While this may not be a politically popular notion, it is not really new. Every issue of nursing's three research journals provides additional evidence of the impact of various nursing interventions on human responses to actual or potential health problems.

The periodic detente between the medical and nursing professions is usually based on a division that proposes that the focus of medical practice should be on cure while the focus of nursing practice should be on care. Unfortunately, the differential definitions of nursing and medical practice are based on political and economic exigencies and have little to do with the real needs of patients. For some patients care and cure are synonymous. For all patients there is a relationship between human responses and actual or potential health problems. In the diagnosis and treatment of human responses, nurses are capable of curing these problems.

REFERENCES

American Nurses' Association. (1980). *Nursing: A social policy statement.* Kansas City, MO: The author.

Barnard, L. (1982). Determining the Focus of Nursing Research, *Maternal Child Nursing, 7*, 299.

Benson, H. (1979). *The mind body effect*. New York: Simon and Schuster.

Brown, B. (1975). *The mind, new body*. New York: Harper & Row.

Cousins, N. (1979). *The anatomy of an illness*. New York: W. W. Norton & Co.

Green, E., & Green, A. (1977). *Beyond biofeedback*. New York: Delta.

Henderson, V. (1961). *Basic principles of nursing care*. London: International Council of Nurses.

Kamiya, J. (1969). Operant control of the EEG alpha rhythm and some of its reported effects on consciousness. In Tart (Ed.), *Altered states of consciousness*. New York: Wiley.

Kamiya, J., Barber, T., Miller, N., Shapiro, D., & Stoyva, J. (Eds.) (1977). *Biofeedback and Self-Control*. Chicago: Aldine Publishing Co.

Lynch, W., & Shuri, U. (1978). Acquired control of peripheral vascular responses. In Schwartz, G., and Shapiro, D. (Eds.), *Consciousness and self-regulation* (Vol. 2). New York: Plenum Press.

Meichenbaum, D. (1977). *Cognitive behavior modification*. New York: Plenum.

Pelletier, K. (1977). *Mind as healer, mind as slayer*. New York: Delta Books.

Roberts, L. Operant conditioning of automatic responses. (1978). Schwartz, G., and Shapiro, D. (Eds.), *Consciousness and self-regulation* (Vol. 2) New York: Plenum Press.

Schwartz, G., & Shapiro, D. (Eds.) (1976–1978). *Consciousness and self-regulation* (2 Vols.). New York: Plenum Press.

Simonton, O., & Simonton, S. (1978). *Getting well again*. Los Angeles: J. P. Tarsher, Inc.